Dave —
In a world with
so much grief, the
world needs people
like you to make
people smile and
laugh & to feel
seen ♡

Michele

Praise for *Your Loss Matters*

"There is nothing harder than going through a life-changing loss and feeling the cold rush of 'woulda, coulda, shoulda'—or worse, people telling you it's time to 'move on.' In *Your Loss Matters*, the permission to be present with whatever comes up is like a breath of fresh air. In a world of 'hurry up and get over it,' having the space and grace to be present with the grief experience is a beautiful and vital healing gift. Michele DeVille understands the nuance and complexity of grief, hitting nearly every angle of the experience. There can never be enough permission slips and validation in the grief journey, and you will want to curl up with a cup of tea, a cozy blanket, and this book."

—**Gina Moffa**, LCSW, grief and trauma therapist
and author of *Moving On Doesn't Mean Letting
Go: A Modern Guide to Navigating Loss*

"Drawing from her own personal experiences with grief, Michele DeVille's words will bring comfort and a deep sense of recognition to anyone grieving. Enormously comforting and validating, *Your Loss Matters* leads readers to a place where their loss is valued, honored, and heard. With loving compassion and heartfelt understanding, Michele has written an honest and easy-to-read book that describes, affirms, and validates the uniqueness of the grief experience. If you find yourself in the midst of grief, this is a must-read to help make sense of it all."

—**Gary Sturgis**, bereavement facilitator and
author of *Surviving Grief: 365 Days a Year*

"Authentic and affirming, *Your Loss Matters* is a wonderful resource for real insights and solace when feeling lost after the death of a loved one. Michele DeVille understands firsthand all the shattered pieces of grief no one wants to face. She presents them in an easy-to-navigate format, providing invaluable insight for profound loss. I will recommend this book to anyone who is searching for wisdom and comfort after loss."

—**Kelly Grosklags**, LICSW, BCD, FAAGC, FT, international speaker, author, and founder of Conversations with Kelly

"Michele DeVille is one of the most skilled writers in the grief and loss space. Her thoughts are beautifully communicated and thought-provoking, and she presents them in a relatable way that allows grievers to feel seen, heard, and validated in all aspects of what they're feeling—even touching on layers of their loss they may not be aware of yet. This book is a valuable, highly needed resource for those who have experienced loss or are journeying through a difficult time. I can't recommend it enough!"

—**Tara Accardo**, founder of Losses Become Gains and podcast host of *Life with Grief*

"From the deep wisdom and lived experience of her own profound loss, Michele DeVille wrote this beautiful book offering readers, particularly those navigating their own heartbreak, a space to feel seen and understood."

—**Meghan Riordan Jarvis**, MA, LCSW, author of *End of the Hour*

"In *Your Loss Matters*, Michele DeVille touches on so many important elements of grief. With short, easy-to-read chapters, she covers important topics including anger and disenfranchised grief, normalizing the grief experience."

—**Lisa Athan**, MA, grief specialist and
executive director of Grief Speaks

"*Your Loss Matters* is a beautiful resource for the grieving. Throughout its pages, Michele DeVille lovingly and tenderly discusses the complicated realities of loss, providing insights into her personal experiences and encouraging the reader to reflect on their own.

Making readers feel validated and seen in their grief, Michele reminds each person that their grief matters and there is no timeline or right or wrong way to navigate loss.

Michele's words are vulnerable and so honestly reflect on the realities of grieving in a society that shies away from the pain of loss. She gives us all a safe space to feel the array of emotions that overwhelm our heart in a time of grief.

The chapters are short and accessible, making it the perfect companion for someone walking through grief. Readers can sit with this book and take their time, reading at a pace that feels right for them. Grief is a personal journey, but books like this feel like a loving friend reaching for our hand, reminding us that there are others who can walk alongside us and provide comfort and connection along the way.

Books like *Your Loss Matters* are such a beautiful gift, showing grieving hearts that they are seen in their sorrow. Her words shine a light into the lonely spaces of grief and honor both love and loss. This book is profound, honest, tender, and hopeful, and I know it will be a blessing to many."

—**Liz Newman**, author of *I Look to the Mourning
Sky* and *I Look to the Gentle Rain*

Your Loss Matters

Real Talk About Grief in a World That Doesn't Get It

Written by
Michele DeVille

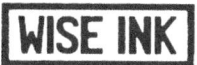

The information shared in this book is a guide offering encouragement,
compassion, validation, and support, but it is not intended to replace the
services of trained mental health professionals nor is it meant to be a substitute
for medical or mental health advice and support. If you are struggling, please
consult with a healthcare professional with regards to your mental health or
physical well-being.

ISBN 13: 978-1-63489-743-3
Library of Congress Catalog Number: 2024921435
Printed in the United States of America
First Printing: 2025
29 28 27 26 25   5 4 3 2 1

Cover design by Emily Mahon
Interior design by Vivian Steckline
Author photo by Jeannine Pohl
Edited by Emily Krempholtz
Proofread by Zenyse Miller and Kerry Stapley
Production editing by Audrey Williams and Hanna Kjeldbjerg

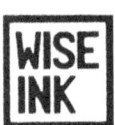 Wise Ink
PO Box 580195
Minneapolis, MN 55458-0195
www.WiseInk.com

Wise Ink is a creative publishing agency for game-changers. Wise Ink authors
uplift, inspire, and inform, and their titles support building a better and more
equitable world. For more information, visit www.WiseInk.com.

To order, visit www.ItascaBooks.com or www.MicheleDeVille.com. Reseller
discounts available.

Contact Michele DeVille at www.MicheleDeVille.com for speaking engage-
ments, freelance writing projects, and interviews.

Mom: This book is for you. Thank you for always being there and for believing in me. Even now, I can feel you cheering me on. I love you.

And to all of my fellow grievers: My heart stands with yours, and I am honored to share this space with you as we continue to walk this life-changing journey together. Your loss and grief matter. Always.

My grief says that I dared to love, that I allowed another to enter the very core of my being and find a home in my heart. Grief is akin to praise; it is how the soul recounts the depth to which someone has touched our lives. To love is to accept the rites of grief.

—Francis Weller

Contents

———————

Introduction

I've always loved writing and have written poetry since I was a young girl. I never dreamed I would be writing a book about loss and grief, yet here I am.

So what led me down the path to writing this book? Life experience, my own personal losses, and a lifelong companion called grief, as well as countless stories of loss, pain, trauma, and grief from so many people. So with nothing but compassion, I wrote this book for you.

I write with the hope it will help you to feel less alone and to create a safe space that encourages you to talk about your pain and what the journey of grief is really like.

We need to change the conversations about loss, pain, and grief. People are hurting everywhere and there will come a time when each and every one of us will experience that first big loss. A significant loss can appear to destroy everything in its path, and can change life as we know it and who we are as a person overnight.

If you're reading this book, you are most likely grieving the loss of someone or something you love. I'm guessing you're in a painful place and fighting to bear what can feel unbearable every day. Or perhaps some time has passed and you're in search of guidance and hope as you continue to integrate loss into your life and move forward while carrying your grief. Regardless of where you are in your own personal grief journey, I get it.

Grief is exhausting and it can feel like your life has been turned inside out—because it has. Even when grief softens (and it will), there will be difficult days ahead.

My heart hurts for the fact that you are in need of this book at all. But I'm also glad that we are connected and that you found your way here.

Loss is part of life and it happens every day. Inevitably, grief will find its way to the door of everyone's heart, yet we live in a society that continues to be uncomfortable with loss, sadness, and grief.

A society that continues to pursue happiness and works hard to bypass pain and misery, regardless of the consequences.

Somehow, grief has become the bad guy. It's viewed as a taboo topic and it really is the big elephant sitting in the middle of the room. Grief is sometimes viewed as an unpleasant, ugly annoyance and one to avoid at all costs. Society urges the grievers of the world to hide it away, get over it, and move on. But grief isn't something to discard or a simple mess to clean up.

Grief is an important journey that requires reflection, soul-searching, and a lot of hard work. When someone in your life dies, everything feels out of sync. Nothing looks familiar and it's easy to feel like you no longer belong or fit in. The truth is, regardless of your best efforts or how much time goes by, grief is often meant to stay.

My first big loss happened when I was just seventeen years old. It was a chilly October night in the fall of my senior year and I was recovering in the hospital from an emergency appendectomy. I heard the sirens late that night, but while I was struggling to sleep with the constant interruptions from the nurses, I was unaware of the tragedy and chaos unfolding just a few miles away.

I will never forget the moment that broke my heart and changed everything. The moment that stripped me of my innocence and changed who I was. My mom walked into my hospital room early Saturday morning and I knew from the look on her face that something was terribly wrong.

With tears in her eyes, she had to tell me my best friend David was dead. The sirens I had heard during the night were the ambulances, police cars, and fire trucks rushing to the scene of an accident that claimed the lives of two young men and injured four others.

David had been killed in a head-on accident. I heard the words but struggled to understand what it meant. How was it possible?

I had just been looking at the proofs of his senior pictures, which were now safely tucked away in a drawer next to my hospital bed.

The room started spinning and I began to sob. The color drained out of my life in that moment, and I would never be the same again.

It was a terrifying, confusing, and lonely time. I went to a very dark place and spent hours writing poetry about death, had thoughts about driving my car off the road so I could be with my friend, and spent many days crying and lying next to his grave at the cemetery. As a young girl, I didn't even know what grief was and I didn't know what to do with the pain.

There were very few resources to help me back then. There were no podcasts, books, support groups, social media accounts, or counselors waiting on Monday to help the students who were grieving such a tragic loss.

I truly felt alone and struggled to find my way back to a life that no longer existed in the same way. I had changed so much that I didn't know who I was anymore. I felt broken and devastated during what was supposed to be one of my most fun and exciting years.

Everything felt overwhelming and I didn't understand that the anger, shame, guilt, shock, sadness, and exhaustion I was feeling was normal. I had no idea that I was grieving nor did I understand grief would become a lifelong companion and play such a big role in who I would become.

I knew how sad I felt at the time, but no one could've told me I would grieve for David for the rest of my life. I still have moments of sadness for him even forty-three years later.

But that's how grief works. Just like love, grief grabs onto your heart and has no intention of letting go. It shifts and changes over time, but if the loss is big enough, it may always be part of you.

Losing David was my first big loss and one I will never forget.

It was a loss that threw me into a dark abyss and I had no tools or resources to help me cope or pull me out.

However, like most people do, I did climb out. While I was no longer the same girl as before, I inched my way back to living life and tried to enjoy my senior year. Moment by moment, I tried to be present and grateful, to find joy while enduring the sadness and pain. It was damn hard, but I learned quickly I had a choice to make. I could let loss destroy me or I could survive. I chose to survive and thrive.

Over the years I would experience many more losses. Losses that broke my heart in ways that couldn't be completely fixed. Losses that would once again throw me into that dark abyss and turn my life upside down. Losses that would leave me feeling misunderstood, isolated, exhausted, and alone.

Not unlike millions of people in the world, I've suffered through several miscarriages, and I've lost best friends and too many family members to count. My dear, sweet mom passed away this past fall, and my first husband Scott, the father of my two oldest daughters, was killed in a tragic boating accident on July 3, 1999. It was an accident that made national headlines and claimed the lives of five young men.

Far too often, we force our grief underground and silence it, because the mere topic of grief feels taboo. I can't tell you how many times I felt alone and judged. I found myself hiding my grief and pretending I was fine when that couldn't have been further from the truth. I wasn't okay, and ignoring my grief and trying to move on without processing every loss made everything far worse. Eventually, numbing out and stuffing my emotions would take a heavy toll. Eventually, my grief would blow up and demand to be felt, seen, and heard.

I didn't know it at the time, but I was learning, evolving, and growing in ways that would carve a path to do this important writing and work. Every loss changed me and brought me one step closer to the person I would become. The person I am today.

I was on a quest to learn everything I could about loss and grief. I took classes, read books, listened to podcasts, studied, and eventually I became a grief educator, specialist, end-of-life doula, and coach. Most importantly, I'm a fellow griever who gets it and understands.

I do this work and write because I don't want anyone else to feel as alone in their grief as I have over the years.

I don't want anyone to feel stuck in the trenches of grief and in desperate need of compassion and support with nowhere to turn. We all need help making sense of the heartbreak, and a reminder we are normal and not crazy.

I've tried to write from the heart. I've tried to tell you the truth about loss from my personal experiences and while you may not always agree, please know my perspectives and the lens from which I view the world has come from my own grief journey as well as the many heartbreaking stories I've witnessed and heard over the years. I don't pretend to have all of the answers, and to be honest, it's challenging writing about a topic that comes with so many different opinions and that everyone will experience differently.

Every class I took and everything I've studied and read has been invaluable and taught me so much, but I've come to realize that all of the training in the world doesn't match the importance of hearing your stories, or my own personal life experience with loss and grief.

While no two losses are the same and everyone will grieve in their own unique way, I too know the struggles of trying to live life after loss.

I've had days when it was challenging to get out of bed. Days when the smallest of tasks felt overwhelming and taking a shower or making a piece of toast felt too hard.

I've had days when I sobbed in the shower or the privacy of my car. Days when I cried so hard and so much, there were no tears left to cry.

There were times when I slept too much and nights when I stared at the ceiling and couldn't sleep at all.

I've had days when I didn't have the energy to focus at work and days when the last thing I felt like doing was a pile of laundry, cooking dinner, or paying the bills.

There were days when everything hurt and I was so distracted by the pain, I couldn't form a full sentence or focus on anything but my grief.

I've had days when I felt shamed, misunderstood, and judged. Days when I felt isolated and alone even when I was surrounded by family and friends.

There were plenty of days when I hid my pain and plastered on fake smiles to cover up my tears. Days when I pretended to be okay when I wasn't okay at all.

But like many grievers, I had to get up every morning and put one foot in front of the other. I had to keep moving. And I did— one small step at a time.

I struggled to navigate through shock, grief, loneliness, and pain as I desperately tried to fit back into a world that didn't always seem to care or understand. I had to relearn how to move forward and try to be the best mom, wife, friend, daughter, and colleague I could be.

It took me a long time to realize that suppressing or dismissing grief comes with consequences that are sometimes hurtful to people, relationships, families, and ourselves.

Pain and grief want us to turn toward it, not run away from it, and when we avoid the pain, it tends to come back.

Grief is demanding. It asks us to surrender and collapse into the endless layers of loss and pain. And as counterintuitive as that may feel, it's when we can wave the white flag and surrender that we move a little closer to hope and to healing some of what feels so broken inside.

There's nothing easy about the grief journey, and in some ways, it's the hardest work you will ever do. A devastating loss will inevitably change the way you view the world and it will force you to relearn how to live when the absence of your loved one presses heavily on your mind and heart.

It's almost like learning to walk again—one painful step at a time. It requires you to relearn how to function in a fast-paced world, dream new dreams, feel safe again, and rebuild what's been destroyed all while honoring your loved one and the past. Sounds easy, right?

Not a chance. It's incredibly hard.

I've come to believe that grievers are some of the most kind and compassionate people I know. Grievers understand how important it is to appreciate life and focus on what matters most. Perspectives change after loss and the grieving tend to see life in a different way.

I don't have all of the answers and this book is not meant to minimize the importance of seeking help if you are feeling stuck. I won't pretend I've personally experienced every kind of loss, because that's simply not true. Nor will I pretend to know the depth of your pain or exactly how you feel, because that's impossible and I'm not walking in your shoes.

But what I do know is that every loss matters and so does your grief.

There's no right, wrong, or perfect way to grieve. I know you didn't ask for any of this, and as grateful as I am for each and every one of you, I wish you didn't have a need for any of these words.

But loss and grief inhabit every corner of the world. People are hurting and grieving behind closed doors and grief lurks in the shadows of our communities, schools, businesses, and homes. We all go to bed at night trusting that we will wake up to experience another day with our loved ones by our side. We leave for school, work, or to enjoy the day with the belief that everyone will return home safe and sound at night.

We have faith that the worst of the storms will pass and the sun will continue to shine. We grow up believing that there is an order to life and feel shocked when the order breaks down, steals our innocence, and turns life inside out.

We believe that parents will always be here to raise their young children, witness their graduations, weddings, and milestones, or become grandparents.

We believe kids will outlive their parents because that's how life's supposed to go.

We believe our friends, siblings, partners, and spouses will be here for the rest of our lives to share a future built on hopes and dreams. Together.

And sadly, we are all lulled into a false sense of security that there will always be more time.

Until there's not. Until the life we believed in and planned on is destroyed in one single moment that changes everything and tears everything apart. Suddenly, the order of how things were supposed to be comes to an abrupt and painful end.

I don't have to tell you how much that sucks and hurts. You're living it right now and my heart aches for you.

Regardless of the loss, you're the only one who can possibly know the depth of your struggles and pain. And as hard as it is, it's so important for you to be honest about your feelings and give your grief a voice.

I can't rescue you or save you from your grief. And as much as I wish I could take your pain away, I can't.

So much of the hard work of grief must be done alone. No one can carry your grief for you, but please know you don't have to walk this painful journey completely by yourself.

My hope is that you will find encouragement, relevance, and love in the pages of this book. I hope you will find companionship, support, and insight as you bravely learn to integrate loss into your new and different life.

Grief is complicated and losing a loved one is one of the hardest things you will ever experience in life. But with time, grief can shift from an uninvited enemy to something you feel more comfortable with. Perhaps a companion of sorts, or even a friend.

Personally, I believe that grief isn't something to get over after a loved one dies. Just like love, the grief you carry in your heart may always remain. But with time, you can move forward and learn to live a full life again.

Human beings have an innate capacity to adapt and survive the most painful of things. You are more resilient than you realize, and that resilience, grace, and courage will help you to survive. The human spirit has the ability to hold on and stay the course even in the wake of life's most powerful and crushing waves.

But part of what it means to survive is finding the courage to keep going and making good choices while trying to discover deeper meaning in life.

You don't have to know all of the answers right now. You will figure it out on your own terms. The answers will reveal themselves when you're ready.

Whether your loss was recent or happened many years ago (and the definition of recent is personal), I've learned that it can be difficult to focus on one thing for long amounts of time after a devastating loss. It can be hard to read a book from front to back when you're exhausted and consumed with grief.

I wrote this book in such a way that you can read the entire book in a day or two, or you can read one chapter at a time. You can pick it up and put it down. You can read and digest it at your own pace. It's a book you can earmark or highlight when you find pages that are relatable to you.

It's a book you can read time and time again and, depending on how you're feeling at the moment, you can refer back to a short chapter that means something to you on a specific day. Certain chapters may feel more relevant in the beginning of your journey and some chapters may be relevant months from now. Last, I want to acknowledge that while many of these chapters are specific to death, every loss matters and much of what I have written about grief can be applied to any type of loss.

This book is written from the heart and every word is written with love from me to you.

I truly hope it reminds you that everything you're feeling and going through is normal and I'm here for you.

Thank you for your courage to open and read the pages in this book. My hope is that it will bring grief into the spotlight and change the way we talk about it just a little bit more. And if these words help you in any way, my heart is full.

Always sending you love, peace, and encouragement. Your grief matters. Always.

—Michele

The Realities of
Loss and Grief

Losing someone you love is brutal and it sucks.

———————————

I will always do my best to offer encouragement but I will never sugarcoat how brutal losing a loved one is.

The pain is agonizing and it can feel as if a hole has been pierced right through your heart.

To lose someone you love is a pain like no other. Life unravels and breaks apart the moment a loved one takes their last breath. And it changes you. You won't be the same person you were before a devastating loss shook up your world, and it's hard to explain that dramatic shift to anyone standing on the other side of your grief. The world around you won't always understand your pain. The loneliness is miserable, and as wrong as it is, grief often goes unacknowledged when you need to feel heard.

No two losses are the same and I can't possibly know what you're feeling right now, but I do understand the pain of grief. I get how lonely and isolated grievers feel. I know how distressing it is to lose someone you care about, and as you carry the immeasurable pain of grief forward, I stand in solidarity with you.

There are no magical words to take your grief away, and honestly, you will always long for your loved one. It is a longing that can't be fulfilled or met. You will miss your person for the rest of your days. You will miss them with every sunrise and every night the sun takes a bow and sets.

You will miss them every day and even though your heart can be reassembled piece by piece, parts will be missing and it won't look quite the same.

On those heavy, grief-filled days, try to soak in the warmth of your memories and honor your loved one in the smallest of ways.

Take good care of yourself and sanction your right to grieve. Don't ignore it. Name your feelings. Own your grief. It's there for a reason and it may not go away.

Losing a loved one is cruel and it's one of the hardest things you will experience in life. I wrote this book for you and I want you to remember your loss matters and your grief deserves respect every single day.

A devastating loss will force you to do a whole lot of things no one wants to do, but you have no other option except to forge on and get things done.

———————————

Losing someone you love is heartbreaking. The loss in and of itself is incredibly hard, but a devastating loss also comes with lots of demands. Demands that require you to do things no one should ever have to worry about or do.

Shortly after someone dies, there are so many decisions and arrangements to make. You're walking around numb and in a fog, yet time keeps marching on and the demands of life force you to keep going regardless of how tired you are.

The reality of loss will often require you to deal with things that should never be asked of anyone.

The first couple of weeks after a life-changing loss are a blur and nothing feels real. You wake up each morning hoping it's just a bad dream but it's not.

Suddenly, grief drains every ounce of energy from you as you struggle to cope with the fallout. As grief takes over, the only thing you want to do is shut yourself away from the pain and try to forget.

But the to-do lists are endless and it doesn't matter how exhausted or heartbroken you are, there are flowers to order, picture boards to create, music to select, and a beautiful service to plan so you can honor your loved one. There are phone calls to make and sometimes, you're forced to have conversations no one wants to have.

Telling my young daughters that their dad died was one of the hardest things I have ever had to do. It crushed me to break their innocent little hearts and tore my own heart right out of my chest.

And let's not forget that the list of things to do doesn't end when the funeral is over and everyone goes home. There are bills to pay, accounts to close, homes to clean out, legal issues to deal with, documents to sign, items to donate, and thank you cards to write. The demands are stressful, and honestly, there will be days when it's hard to get out of bed let alone deal with an endless series of tasks you have no choice but to do.

After my first husband Scott died, I was so overwhelmed. The week of the funeral was a blur. I was worried about my little girls. The phone never stopped ringing and there were reporters wanting an interview. I needed to deal with the coroner and make calls I didn't want to make. I had to pick out clothes for him to wear and decide if it was going to be an open or closed casket.

There was an estate to deal with and although we were divorced and I had just remarried, we still owned the house together, so I was charged with going through all of his stuff and getting the house ready to sell. There were bills to pay, accounts to close, documents to sign, items to donate, and hundreds of wedding *and* funeral thank you notes to write all at the same time. Not to mention I had a new husband to worry about in the middle of the chaos.

I had to deal with lawsuits for over a year. I was exhausted and to make it worse, I felt alone. Because Scott and I were no longer married, I felt like I had to hide my grief. It broke me in ways that are still difficult to talk about.

It was a stressful time for all of us and the concern for my little girls was constantly on my mind.

I learned the hard way that it's important to take good care of yourself in the early days of grief. Listen to your body and if you're feeling overloaded, take a step back and try to get some well-deserved rest. Make sure you're staying hydrated and don't forget to eat. Try to move your body in the smallest of ways and get outside for fresh air.

Easier said than done, right? I get it, but grief can feel like a full-time job and it's important to take care of your mind, body, and heart as you struggle to do everything that's being asked of you.

There will be days when you can't possibly do it all. Days when the load you're trying to carry is too much and you need help. Don't be afraid to ask for help or reach out to someone if you just need to talk. I talked to anyone who would listen back then, even if it was my hairstylist or massage therapist. There are people who will understand all of this because they have walked the same path as you. People who will show up and want to help you.
I know how overwhelming life can feel after a devastating loss and I know there are things you don't want to do.

Be gentle with all that feels so broken right now, and when life is demanding too much from you, don't be afraid to set a boundary or two. You may not feel like it today, but you're amazing. Please know I see your grief and I'm proud of you.

It's impossible to go back to a place that no longer exists. A place that was forever altered when loss shattered everything and turned life upside down. The only direction is forward while trying to learn how to exist in the world without your loved one — and that's a difficult thing to do.

―――――――――――――

One of the most challenging things for anyone facing the devastation of loss is desperately trying to find a way back to how things were before.

But the truth is, there's no finding your way back to before. Loss changes so many things and as much as people wish they could get back to normal, life doesn't feel normal or look the same.

There's no going back to what was. The only option is to dig deep to find the courage to move forward into the unknown.

There are no shortcuts as you stumble forward with so many unanswered questions, and it's scary to live life with the uncertainty that comes with loss.

There will be days when you feel like you're spinning around in circles, stuck, and going nowhere. Those days are unsettling, and it's easy to feel like you will never find a way out of the messy maze of loss and grief. A maze that's trapped you and is standing in the way of you moving toward better and brighter days. But you can. One step at a time.

I know it's painful to accept that your life is forever altered and to know you can never go back. The same exact life you lived before is over and as difficult as it is, you must now find ways to build a different one.

It takes time to rebuild in a world you no longer recognize, but with patience and courage you will slowly transition into a new way of being—and honestly, that takes guts.

Don't let fear stand in the way of moving forward. Have faith that you will grow around the grief. With that growth, life will become full of possibilities. Stay the course, and eventually, you will find your way.

Grief doesn't negotiate and it shows up whether you're ready for it or not. Grief moves in and often has no intention of leaving. Perhaps it's supposed to stay after someone you love dies, and because of love, grief rarely compromises.

There are many things that can be negotiated in life. We, as human beings, can often push back and try to work on finding different outcomes or solutions when something doesn't work or feel right.

But grief isn't one of them. Grief doesn't negotiate and as much as it would be nice to find a different solution after a life-changing loss, grief has a mind of its own. Without compromise, it will show up and make itself right at home.

Loss happens every day. And where you find loss you will find grief. It's impossible to avoid or negotiate it away. Grief doesn't operate like that. If the loss is big enough, grief becomes a constant companion as you push your way through the mess.

It's true that grief won't always be so bold, loud, and intense. There will be days when it quietly hums in the background as the sharp edges of grief dull.

But it's always there, poised and ready to be heard when the tough days hit or unexpected grief bombs go off and knock you down.

Nothing about heartbreaking loss is easy and sometimes it can feel like grief has taken over every part of you, emotionally, mentally, and physically.

With that being said, there will also be days when the waves of pain subside and you will find the courage to swim back to the surface of your life to catch your breath.

There will be days when it doesn't feel as difficult to face the day or get out of bed. And when the waters calm, it will be possible to find a splash or two of joy.

I know it's hard and I know it can feel like nothing will ever feel right in your world again.

But it can.

The gaps between bad and good days will get longer and just like the seasons, grief will shift and change. The sun will shine, the leaves will change colors, the snow will melt, and the flowers will grow and bloom again. Nothing stays exactly the same and you can grow and bloom again too.

You can't force the good days to come but it's my hope you will eventually feel more love than pain. Grief may always live in your heart, but it's here for a reason, and one of those reasons, my grieving friend, is love.

Home is where the heart is but when your heart breaks from a life-shattering loss, it's hard to feel at home anywhere.

––––––––––––––––

I don't know that I've ever felt as homesick as I did after my mom died. Something shifted in me that day, and a part of me died on the inside.

While I hadn't physically lived with my parents for many years, part of my forever home disappeared when she died.

I'm sure you've heard the expression, "Home is where the heart is." Even though it's a lovely thought, it's hard to feel at home anywhere when your heart is shattered and broken in two.

A home is supposed to be a place that offers refuge, safety, and comfort. It's a place to return to even when life has temporarily stolen the light away and everything feels gloomy and dim.

Even as an adult, I felt like an orphan. Losing my mom left a huge hole in my heart. I felt lost and disoriented with no place for my grief to go.

Unsettled, I struggled to find my place in this new and different world. I lost my mom, my emotional lifeline, my biggest supporter and friend. I lost part of my identity and a very important role. If I was no longer a daughter or caretaker, who was I now?

It's true that a significant loss tosses life up in the air and you never know what it will look like when all of the pieces land on the ground. It's often a tangled mess and it can be quite overwhelming to try and patch all those broken pieces back together again.

How do you find peace when living in the tension of the bittersweet? It's a place that holds so many memories yet feels so empty at the same time. A place that used to ring with your loved one's laughter but now holds a deafening silence that only you can hear.

There are no easy answers and the journey to get back "home" is hard. The truth is, home may never feel the same, but that doesn't mean you can't rebuild your life and a new place called home.

It won't be easy, that much I know. But it's possible, and finding a renewed sense of purpose in your life is a good place to begin.

Things have drastically changed since my mom died, but with intention, I have filled my heart and home with memories of my mom and it helps me to feel closer to her even though she's gone.

I will always be her daughter and she will always be my mom. I may not be able to see her, but I talk to her every day. And you can do the same.

I'm sorry your heart is broken and you're struggling to find your way back home. Eventually, you will find your way forward. When you do, you won't feel as homesick as you do right now.

Loss isn't something you can completely prepare for. When a loved one dies, it's hard to know what to do and it's even harder to know how to grieve.

———————————

Everyone will grieve in their own personal way. Grief is as unique as our fingerprints and there is no one way to do it right. After all, do any of us truly know how to grieve?

When loss hits, it rearranges everything and turns life inside out. It's impossible to completely prepare for all that comes with a loss that shatters your heart and world into a million little pieces.

Grief isn't something that can be easily mastered, and it's not something you become good at. Grief is complicated and it doesn't follow a straight line. It's messy, unpredictable, and never stays the same.

There's no way to avoid it and even if you've grieved before, grief can change course and look different with every new and devastating loss.

Grievers constantly tell me they don't know what to do with their grief. They struggle to know how to grieve and question if they are doing it right. People often worry they won't survive and the unrealistic expectations of others don't help.

Honestly, there were times in my life I didn't even know I was grieving because I didn't know what grief was.

Perhaps grief isn't something people are supposed to know how to do but rather it's something to experience as it unfolds with each and every loss. Perhaps it's not something to "get through" but instead it's something you must learn to manage and carry forward.

The truth is, you will experience grief after a significant loss. And until grief shows up at your own door, it's impossible to truly prepare for it or understand just how challenging it can be. However, you can develop skills to help you better navigate grief and there are many resources and tools that you can draw upon with each and every loss you encounter in life.

Grief has no set agenda. It doesn't expect you to have all the answers in the beginning, nor do you have to figure everything out today. Grief will slowly reveal itself to you and it's possible to grow with and around your grief over time. You may be a different person now, and life may not be the same, but it's entirely possible to live with loss and discover new ways to enjoy beautiful moments in life again.

If you're trying to carry the heavy, somewhat clunky, and uncomfortable weight of grief on your weary shoulders, you deserve credit for the hard work you're doing every single day.

You don't have to know exactly how to grieve but it's important to recognize it and acknowledge it. Grief is part of you now and you will learn how to live with it—no grief expertise required.

A life filled with grief is like a jigsaw puzzle that can never be put back together in the same way as before. Pieces of the puzzle are missing and it forces you to relearn how to live in the world knowing pieces of your life are gone forever and can't be replaced.

———————————

A devastating loss will test you in unexpected ways and sometimes it will test your will to keep going and survive. Grief quickly becomes part of your daily life and it's like a jigsaw puzzle that can't be completed because pieces are scattered everywhere.

Loss forces people to relearn how to live and exist in a world that feels unfamiliar. The pain of knowing pieces of your life are gone forever and can't be replaced is difficult to accept and chips away at your heart.

The feelings of isolation and abandonment are hard to describe, and to relearn how to function in life after loss takes resilience and time.

It's exhausting to learn how to act in the world when your life has changed because of a loss that's left you feeling broken on the inside and has stolen important pieces of your life story. Pieces you can't get back.

It's no wonder people feel hopeless and come to believe they are forever destined to live a life of sorrow and suffering.

I remember going back to school just days after my best friend David died in a car accident. Everything seemed different and I felt like a stranger wandering listlessly through the hallways that once brought me comfort and joy.

I wanted to scream at people laughing in the lunchroom or chatting about ridiculous things that no longer mattered to me. How could they be laughing when a friend and fellow student was dead? Didn't anyone understand the enormity of what just happened? Didn't they understand that life would never be the same?

But that's what happens in the world after loss. People quickly go back to their lives even though you feel stuck in quicksand, unable to think or move. The world feels terrifying and no longer makes sense.

It's maddening, really, and it can feel impossible to fit in no matter where you go or how hard you try.

A heartbreaking loss shatters our illusions of safety and control. It robs people of a sense of security and leaves people feeling vulnerable and afraid.

I was terrified for months after David died. The promise of immortality and the innocence of youth had been shattered and was nowhere to be found. My world no longer felt safe.

My life and the grief I carried was like a jigsaw puzzle. Key pieces of who I was and all I had loved were missing, and even at the age of seventeen, I knew some of those pieces were gone and couldn't be replaced. I didn't know how to live in the world anymore. I no longer fit in.

An unraveling of your daily life happens quickly in the wake of loss and it can feel as if you've been banished to an island of despair, isolated and alone.

Believe me when I say I get it. I understand how easy it is to slip into a place where hope is nowhere to be found.

But with time and effort, you can carve out a new path in life and relearn how to exist in the world. Piece by piece, you will learn to patch your broken heart and life back together again. It will look different and you will be forever changed, but it's possible to claw your way through the darkness and emerge into a world that inspires you to find hope and light again. Death is permanent but losing hope is temporary—and thank God for that.

Progress is both slow and subtle, but your grief will change, your heart will continue to beat, and the sun will shine again.

A different version of your puzzle can be put back together, even though pieces will always be missing and the whole may never look quite the same. You've got this.

It can take years to adapt and step into a new way of living after the devastation of loss destroys so much in life. Trying to relate to a world that doesn't slow down for anyone or anything can make it even harder to rise above the ruins.

_____

Everything looks different after loss barges in and tears down the walls of your life. Suddenly, the world you're trying so hard to live and breathe in doesn't look the same anymore. And in some ways it will never look the same again.

The heartbreak of loss changes life in irreversible ways and it can make you feel like your life is in ruins.

Understandably, one of the biggest questions grievers ask is, "How do I adapt to living life in a world that doesn't always get it or slow down for anyone?"

Grief will quickly throw you into unfamiliar territory and there will be moments when you feel like the life you once knew is nothing more than a distant memory.

It's disturbing to wake up each morning knowing that, for you, life is different now and there's no going back. Finding the courage to move forward every day can be overwhelming and overloaded with uncertainty and fear.

To be frank, it's hard to keep up the pace with a world that thrives on staying as busy as possible and has no intention of slowing down for you and your grief. As you desperately try to function while under duress, it can feel like a clear line has been drawn in the sand between "your world" and "their world."

The people who casually observe your sorrow but fail to understand it will encourage you to move on quickly because they need you to adapt and rejoin their world again.

But their world didn't just collapse and, unlike you, the people in your life are not fighting to exist in a world that's stretched beyond recognition and no longer makes sense. A world full of unanswered questions, heartbreak, and pain.

It's unreasonable to expect you to see the world in the same way as before. The lines between the before and after are muddy and it's emotionally and physically draining to keep crossing back and forth between the two.

It can feel like you're suspended in between two worlds for a very long time. The world before death ripped it apart and the different world you're trying to live in after grief knocked at your door, and without an invitation, moved right in.

It's important to protect your heart as you try to find ways to adapt to life after loss. To walk gently as you learn how to avoid the many land mines that come with grief.

The train of grief has no final destination and it will depart in and out of your heart time and time again. You may feel better and even try to get off the train once in a while, but inevitably there will be more difficult days ahead. Even though the intensity of grief fades, you may always be a passenger on this wildly imperfect ride.

Don't get discouraged. You will learn to unpack some of the heavy baggage of loss and, yes, it's possible to rejoin "their world" as you find ways to rebuild and rise above the ruins.

You can't wish grief away, cry it away, exercise it away, or eat and drink it away. It will continue to lurk in the shadows, and as difficult as it is, you can learn to carry your grief forward and somehow survive a loss that changed your life in the most unimaginable of ways.

Where there's loss, there will be grief. You can't escape the grip of grief, especially when the deep bond of love exists. The greater the love, the greater the grief. It's both a beautiful and heartbreaking part of being human.

A devastating loss and the grief that accompanies it is a challenge. There will be days when it feels like there's no way to move forward, let alone experience good moments again. Days when you have lost your sense of direction and question how you will find your way through it and survive.

There will be days when grief consumes you and it will be hard to focus on anything but the excruciating pain. Days when your ability to function or process what happened is heavily compromised.

Yet we live in a world that doesn't always understand just how difficult loss really is. People standing on the outside of your grief can't relate and society is unfair when it comes to expecting grievers to hide their pain and move on.

But it's not that simple. Grief never is. It can be a complicated and grueling journey that demands you survive things you never thought you could.

Hiding the pain doesn't help grievers to adapt or move forward in life at all. Avoidance does nothing but encourage the pain to fester and grow. It makes everything worse because suppressed pain doesn't go away. Instead, it manifests in unhealthy ways.

Society uses happiness as a marker to gauge how well you're doing and people have been conditioned to believe that struggling, grieving, and pain are bad. We live in a culture that believes positivity is the answer to all of our problems and even applauds people who pull up their big-kid pants and move beyond the tough stuff that happens in life.

As much as the rest of the world wants you to get over it, you can't wish the pain of grief away. You can't cry it away, eat it away, exercise it away, or drink it away. You can't work it away, outrun it, or find a magical cure.

Grief isn't going anywhere. It's important to face your undigested pain or it will continue to gnaw away at your heart.

Choosing to sit with your grief is one of the only ways to lessen the pain. And while it's necessary to clear the way for moments of happiness and joy, it can be difficult to feel positive and look to the future in the early days, weeks, and months.

There's nothing easy about what's been asked of you, especially when you're trying to find solid ground to stand on after the world shifted and gave way beneath your feet.

But pain needs space to stretch out and unfold. It takes courage to sit inside of your pain, and grief doesn't exist in the magical Land of Oz. You can't click your heels and wish your way back to the life you lived before.

I wish you could wish your pain away but it's best to stay away from unhealthy coping tools. Instead, accept the unspoken invitation to meet your grief face-to-face. Trying to numb the pain with food, alcohol, drugs, or sex will do more damage than good. I've tried to numb my grief many times over the years, and it didn't work.

It's important to engage with grief and allow all of your emotions to move through you so they don't overwhelm you or set you back.

Life won't always feel this hard and things can get better, but it will take hard work, a willingness to address the pain, and acceptance of how different your life has become.

As time unfolds, it's my wish that some of what looks and feels so different will lead you to discover meaning, purpose, and joy.

You can do this.

It's hard to accept the unacceptable. The knowing that your person will never walk through the door again or give you a hug that you so badly need. The knowing that regardless of how much time goes by, grief has become part of who you are.

———————————

I'm sorry if the words I write resonate with you. I wish none of it was true. I wish I could make it better and take every ounce of your pain away.

But I can't. The only thing I can do is continue to offer love, support, and the truth as I have come to know it.

I have learned that accepting the unacceptable is one of the most difficult things anyone will have to do. It hurts to know that no matter how much you long to change what happened, you can't.

Accepting the unacceptable when grieving a monumental loss can leave you feeling powerless. The yearning for what was is all-consuming at times and in those moments, it can feel as if grief has taken control over every part of you and your life.

Acceptance is a big, bold, complicated word in the world of grief. But it's an important part of the process and it's necessary if you want to heal and move forward in life.

I understand that accepting the unacceptable may feel impossible right now. I get it. I really do. And perhaps there are certain things you will never fully accept even though you know them to be painfully true.

It's my sincere hope that you will continue to find ways to live and grow around the grief that has become such a big part of you.

It's my hope you can slowly learn to accept the smallest of things when you're ready, so the chains of grief don't keep you stuck and render you powerless.

While it may be challenging to accept a tragic loss in the beginning, you can always start with accepting the tangled emotions that seem to constantly bombard your heart. You can learn to accept how you feel and this can empower you to keep moving after loss.

Nothing about loss and grief is easy. I know how heavy and exhausting it can feel, and I know the desperation of wanting to see your loved one walk through the door. I know the helplessness of yearning for the chance to say "I love you" one more time or feel those warm hugs you miss so much and can no longer share.

Be gentle with your heart. Never stop giving yourself grace and don't try to push the pain away or skip ahead of what grief will ask of you. It's difficult to mend all that feels so broken if you don't allow yourself to feel.

Try to do at least one kind thing for yourself every day and find someone you can rely on who will be here for you.

Don't give up. As the road of grief unfolds and reveals itself to you, be patient with yourself as you try to accept even the tiniest parts of what feels so unacceptable to you. There will be days when it feels like there's no pause button when it comes to grief. Days when as much as you would like to, it's impossible to leave it at home. The truth is, grief often travels with you wherever you go. It would be nice if you could flip a switch and, when it hurts too much, turn off the pain. But it's not that simple. You're doing the best you can in an unimaginable situation you didn't ask to be in.

———————————

Human beings need to feel a sense of control in their daily lives, and thankfully, we have the power of choice in so much of what we do.

But loss is often out of our control and rarely would anyone ever choose to walk the road of grief.

Nonetheless, grief is part of life. There's no choice when it comes to grieving a heartbreaking loss and whether you like it or not, grief will find you.

Of course it would be nice if you could hit a pause button in the middle of the pain. It would be nice if grief could be controlled with a remote and completely turned off for a while.

But there's no easy way to turn grief off and on at will. Grief doesn't care if it shows up at the most inconvenient of times. And when it does, it won't matter what you're doing, where you are, or what day of the week it is. You can have the best of intentions about having fun at a family gathering, participating in a social event, or putting your best foot forward at work. But sometimes the best of intentions fall short. There will be times when grief is difficult to control and, whether it's convenient or not, will demand to be seen and heard.

And that's okay. You don't always have to hide your grief or try to rein it in.

There will be days when it doesn't feel safe to share your feelings with the outside world. Days when you don't have the capacity to express your pain out loud. There will be those moments when it feels safer to excuse yourself and grieve in silence instead of sharing your pain with someone.

So what do you do when you don't have the capacity to deal with or share your grief?

Remember, this is your personal journey, and while grief may not have an automatic pause button, it is possible to take a break from the pain.

Engage in activities that can break up your negative thoughts, even if it's only for five minutes.

Get your nails or hair done. Go shopping. Meet a friend for lunch or get outside for a walk. Take a yoga class or catch a new movie at the theater. Organize a closet or volunteer your time.

It's okay to have an unraveling kind of day, but know that a little bit of distraction can go a long way. Human beings have the instinctive capacity to adapt and survive.

You didn't choose this path, and you certainly didn't choose the heartbreak of a devastating loss, but you can choose how to grieve. Be gentle with your heart. When the downpours of grief come, let them wash over you and remember, it's okay to take a break once in a while and find shelter from the rain.

There will always be dreaded
milestones to get through in the
journey of grief. Milestones that
bring extra pain and are difficult
to get through and overcome. But
in the beginning, every day can
feel like a milestone and it takes
courage to keep going when it feels
much easier to retreat and hide.

———————————

If the loss is big enough, the journey of grief can last forever—and
when trying to function in the world without your loved one, forever can feel like a really long time. Because it is.

The first year or two are filled with potholes and as hard as it is,
many of the potholes are lying in wait and difficult to avoid.

Life is full of milestones that celebrate so many wonderful
things. We live in a world that celebrates the special occasions in
life and whether it's a birthday, graduation, wedding, anniversary,
or the holidays, people look forward to the milestones that bring
happiness and joy. Until they don't.

A heartbreaking loss changes so many things in life and one of
the many things lost along the way is the ability to find the same
joy on those special days you used to look forward to and love.

The milestones in life can come with conflicting emotions and
dread. And to celebrate in the same way as before can be difficult
when grief is in the air and your loved one is no longer able to
celebrate by your side.

Society won't always understand and sometimes people will
urge you to cheer up, celebrate, and have fun. But it's hard to cele-

brate days that no longer hold quite the same meaning as they did before loss tarnished so many things.

Milestones are hard. Don't feel bad if you're struggling and, in some ways, fear those extra-hard days. It's normal and there's nothing wrong with you.

It's perfectly fine if you don't feel like celebrating or if you need to shed a few tears. The rest of the world may need you to "be yourself" but it's more important that you honor your feelings and your grief. This isn't about society; it's about you.

Sometimes the anticipation of the milestone is worse than getting through the actual day itself and it can leave you feeling on edge. Nonetheless, whether the days before are harder or the day itself knocks you down, it's possible to get through the difficult milestones, especially with a plan. Sometimes you might even surprise yourself and enjoy the day.

Please take care of your heart on the tough milestone days and remember, every day can feel like a milestone to survive in the early days after loss.

We spend far too much time trying to make sense out of something that will never make sense to our broken hearts. There will never be a good enough reason or a comforting answer to the why. How could there be when someone you love is gone and loss took some of the best parts of your life away?

———————————

Human beings are curious by nature. We have a need to find answers and understand the why behind so many of the things that happen in life. We try to make sense out of everything and it's natural to want to believe there's a reason for it all.

But that doesn't work so well when it comes to a devastating, soul-crushing loss. A loss that shakes everything up and breaks your heart.

It's true that we grieve many difficult losses because of love, but that's also why grief is so painful and hard. And that's why losing someone you love deeply may never make sense to your wounded heart.

The phrase "everything happens for a reason" rarely brings comfort when people are thrown into the bottomless pit of loss. What possible reason could fill the huge void after someone you love dies?

There are no answers that will be good enough when you lay awake at night struggling to make sense of a loss that stripped you of the life you loved so much.

I have heard it all and I'm sure you have too: Everything happens for a reason. They are in a better place. Someday you will know the why and find the answers you're desperately searching for.

Honestly, so much of what's said to grievers is meaningless and most of the time, the words simply don't help.

Losing someone you love is one of the most painful, cruel, and heartbreaking things people will go through. You are left with an ache that can't be calmed and there is no good enough reason for the gaping hole in your life.

There's a reason for your grief but there will rarely be a good enough reason that justifies the why or brings relief.

I'm sorry you're carrying the weight of loss and hurting so much. I really am. It's hard to carry the truth of just how devastating your loss is for one day, yet alone for a lifetime.

My heart hurts for you, and please know you don't have to do this completely alone. And on the days when you can't stop searching for the answers that never seem to come, focus on the love. Because sometimes love is the only thing people have to cling to in the middle of the chaos.

You will miss your loved one for the rest of your life, but you will also grieve for all of the things your loved one is missing. "They should be here" can easily become a constant thought playing over and over again in your mind.

_____

There's a deep longing that comes with loss. A longing for what was and what was supposed to be. A yearning for your loved one as well as your old self.

But people also grieve for all of the things their loved one is missing out on. Both the most ordinary of things and the big events in life can stir up grief, and the nagging feeling of "they should be here" never goes away.

They should be here to see their children or grandchildren grow up.

They should be here for their daughter's wedding and to walk her down the aisle.

They should be here to celebrate graduation with all of their friends, go to college, get married, and have a family of their own.

They should be here to go on that trip you always dreamed about.

Honestly, there are so many things your loved one will never get to experience and the pain of knowing your loved one is missing out on so many amazing things runs deep and wide.

I try to bring my loved one's presence into so much of what I experience in life. To honor them and stay connected when the "they should be here" hits and breaks my heart all over again.

But I know it's not the same and I understand the grief you

feel every time you remember your loved one is missing something they should be here for.

Grace. Grace. Grace. Allow yourself to feel every emotion when they come flooding in. Dare to grieve and find special ways to honor your loved one when you feel their absence the most.

Talk about your pain. Share your loved one's name. Tell their story. Look at the pictures. Plant a tree in their memory. Wear their favorite hat, T-shirt, or piece of jewelry. Listen to their favorite music or cook their favorite meal.

There's nothing easy about loss, and while grief is here for a reason, the journey is long and hard. Be kind to yourself and tend to your wounds.

You're loved and your grief matters. You're grieving because someone you love should be here and when they are missing out on the things they would've loved, it hurts.

Similar to the changing of seasons, grief changes and shifts. But as beautiful as each season can be, it can bring painful reminders of what no longer is.

––––––––––––––––––

As I write this, fall is in the air. Fall has always been my favorite season and one I look forward to. Living in the Midwest comes with crisp fall mornings and stunning colors as the leaves begin to change.

By the time September rolls around each year, I'm more than ready for the cooler weather, football, and wearing sweaters and jeans.

Honestly, I love all of the seasons but sometimes the changing of seasons is difficult. Minnesota winters can be brutal, snowy, and bitterly cold.

Nonetheless, the seasons shift and change every year and I always think about how similar the journey of grief can be. Grief shifts and changes. It ebbs and flows. And if you look hard enough, you can discover moments of beauty, even though the many seasons of grief can come with undeniable sadness and pain.

And the changing of the seasons, regardless of where you live, can stir up your grief and remind you of all you've lost.

It can be as simple as remembering picking apples with your loved one on a cool fall day, trick or treating, or taking a drive on a Sunday afternoon to enjoy the beautiful leaves.

It can be as simple as making snow angels on a snowy winter day, going skating, drinking hot chocolate, or baking cookies.

It can be a warm memory of planting tulips in early spring or going out for a walk once the snow melts and the trees magically turn green.

It can be wearing flip-flops and shorts on a hot summer day, running through freshly cut grass, or watching the fireworks on the Fourth of July.

Whatever it is, the seasons can stir up bittersweet memories and in turn, stir up your grief, no matter how long it's been.

My mom loved watching football. She loved to wear her favorite color purple and cheer for the Vikings, her favorite team. Watching the Vikings now that she's gone is tough. It makes me smile as I think about her but it also comes with tears and wishing she were here.

The changing of the seasons is part of life and so is the grief you now carry in your heart. Don't push it away. Let it unfold. Sit inside of the change. Experience it. Feel it. Surrender to it. Choose to embrace life again.

And on those days when your grief and all of the change is just too much, hold on to the love. Regardless of the season, love is in the air.

**Relationships change in unexpected
ways after a devastating loss. It can
feel like a difficult loss shatters
everything, and sometimes, the
people you thought would weather
the darkest of storms with you
disappear when you need them most.**

––––––––––––––

A soul-shattering loss quickly pushes grief into the spotlight. I've learned there's nothing like grief when it comes to shaking up and changing support systems or, worse yet, tearing relationships apart.

Sometimes, the foundation of relationships cracks and the emotional lifelines you so badly need fray and fall apart. Feeling abandoned by the people you thought you could count on can come as quite a shock.

Honestly, losing the support of family, friends, and colleagues hurts, and it's understandable if you feel confused, dismissed, and alone.

I know it's hard but it's important to remember that people don't always deal with the tough stuff in life very well. People cope in different ways and as hard as it is to accept, not everyone will be prepared to sit with you inside the uncomfortable or bear witness to your pain.

Some people will find a way to adapt and grow alongside you in this new chapter of your life, but many won't.

Grievers are often surprised when the people they thought would walk through the fires with them fall silent and disappear. On the contrary, it can be a pleasant surprise when people you barely know show up and support you through the most challenging times of your life.

Unfortunately, society is uncomfortable with grief. The people in our lives don't always know what to do or say after loss tears life apart. People often stumble carelessly through their words, dishing out platitudes while hoping they will help your pain magically disappear. And as difficult as it is, some will turn their backs on you and walk away.

Relationships will change and I know this can feel like another loss that adds more layers of grief to your bruised and battered heart. But you're not obligated to maintain a relationship with anyone who is draining your energy or making you feel worse.

Loss will change your perspective in unexpected ways, and the grieving often see life through a completely different lens. Sometimes, letting a relationship fall away is for the best.

Grievers don't have the time and energy to deal with more disappointment or drama after a life-changing loss. Tolerance wanes and when support systems let grievers down, some relationships will break, regardless of how strong that bond may have been in the past.

When family and friends don't seem to understand the gravity of your pain, it can feel exhausting to keep investing in relationships that take more than they give.

The truth is, the world doesn't owe you anything and not everyone in your life will get it or understand. Not everyone has the emotional capacity to meet you where you are in your grief.

I would like to believe that people have the best intentions and perhaps they want to help but simply don't know how. That's when we need to give the gift of grace to them and ultimately to ourselves.

It's not your job to please everyone and it's okay to move forward and cut ties even if it means leaving a relationship behind.

What's most important is that you take care of yourself and

have your own back. And sometimes taking care means trusting yourself enough to let a relationship go and saying goodbye to someone adding to your pain.

This is your journey and you're the only one who can decide when it's time to let go. But whether you hold on or find the courage to cut ties, it's healing to forgive and we are all trying to find our way through the muddy waters of grief.

Don't settle for less or feel like you're asking for too much. You deserve to have people in your life who will continue to show up and embrace you with unconditional love, compassion, and support.

A devastating loss changes you in unimaginable ways. Loss strips part of your identity away, and it can feel as if the person you once were disappeared into thin air. It can take a long time to figure out who you are and who you will become after loss crushes your heart. The relationship you have with yourself changes, and it can be a long path of discovery in a world that wants you to be the same person you were before. Don't let the expectations of others dictate who you are today or who you will become. This is your grief journey, and you need to give yourself grace as you struggle to pick up the pieces and carve out a different but meaningful life.

A significant loss can bring life as you know it to an abrupt halt. In the beginning, nothing looks or feels quite the same.

Inevitably, loss changes people, and perhaps it's supposed to. It's impossible to be the exact same person you were before loss turned your life upside down.

I remember everything about the moment I was told my best friend David had died. Suddenly, a harsh line was drawn and etched into my heart, clearly dividing my life into the before and after. One single moment in time changed my young seventeen-year-old self forever.

Instantaneously, a flicker of denial appeared as the life I knew and trusted flashed before my eyes and then disappeared. I remember what it was like to feel the innocence of youth drain out of my body as I screamed and burst into tears.

My heart broke that day, yet I lacked the ability to comprehend what had just happened to my best friend whom I had loved since first grade. I certainly didn't understand how different my life would be.

It's impossible for things to stay exactly the same after loss, and in the beginning, the shock consumes you and it's difficult to truly understand just how much life's about to change.

But change is imminent on the heels of loss. Once grief burrows its way deep inside your heart, you won't know how to be the person you were just seconds before loss flattened you.

On occasion, you might catch a glimpse of a dim version of yourself, but parts of you will be unrecognizable and you won't be the same. Yet the world around you remains unscathed by a loss that paralyzed parts of you. It is a world that somehow needs and expects everything to go back to normal when your normal is nowhere to be found.

Sadly, these unrealistic expectations put pressure on the grieving. Pressure to move on. Pressure to be okay when you're not. Pressure to be someone who no longer exists in the same way.

This doesn't work in grief. People change and the relationship you have with yourself changes in deep and profound ways. It can be a challenge to figure out who you are and who you will become in the early days, weeks, and months after loss. Honestly, it's a bit unnerving when you don't recognize parts of yourself in the mirror.

But here's the thing. You don't have to find all the answers or figure out who you will become right now. You are not obligated to be someone you're not, nor do you have to paste a thick layer of positivity over your sadness and hide your grief.

You've been thrown into a world of chaos you didn't ask to be in and it's no wonder you feel lost and numb. How is anyone supposed to know who they are after a devastating loss has rearranged life from the inside out?

It takes time and self-awareness, but eventually, the thick fog will clear. Slowly you will emerge and, while different, you will begin to recognize both old and new pieces of yourself inside of your grief.

You will learn to grow around the loss and the grief you now carry. You won't be the same exact person as before, but with patience and self-love, you will begin to feel more comfortable with your new, grieving self.

For now, it's okay to feel unsteady as you try to settle into the unfamiliar. It's okay to stumble as you try to find your way forward in a life that continues to unfold in unpredictable ways.

The death of a loved one doesn't have to be the end of your story. With time, you will find the courage to write new chapters as you discover ways to find meaning and purpose again. You won't constantly feel like you're sitting on top of a cliff waiting for grief to consume every part of you and pull you over the edge.

It took a long time for me to find myself after David died. But with hope, patience, and determination, I learned how to live a full life again even though I was a different person and grief remained in my heart.

Is it easy? Absolutely not. Does it happen overnight? No. Will you have setbacks and days when your grief is so loud it's hard to think clearly or focus on anything else? Yes.

But there will come a time when the dust settles and you can wipe away the fog in the mirror and find clarity again.

It may not always feel like it but I want you to know it's possible for joy to coexist with your grief. It's possible to laugh despite the many tears that fall. It's possible to recover and reclaim pieces of yourself you thought were forever lost while discovering beautiful pieces of the amazing person you will become.

You are loved for who you were, who you are, and who you will become.

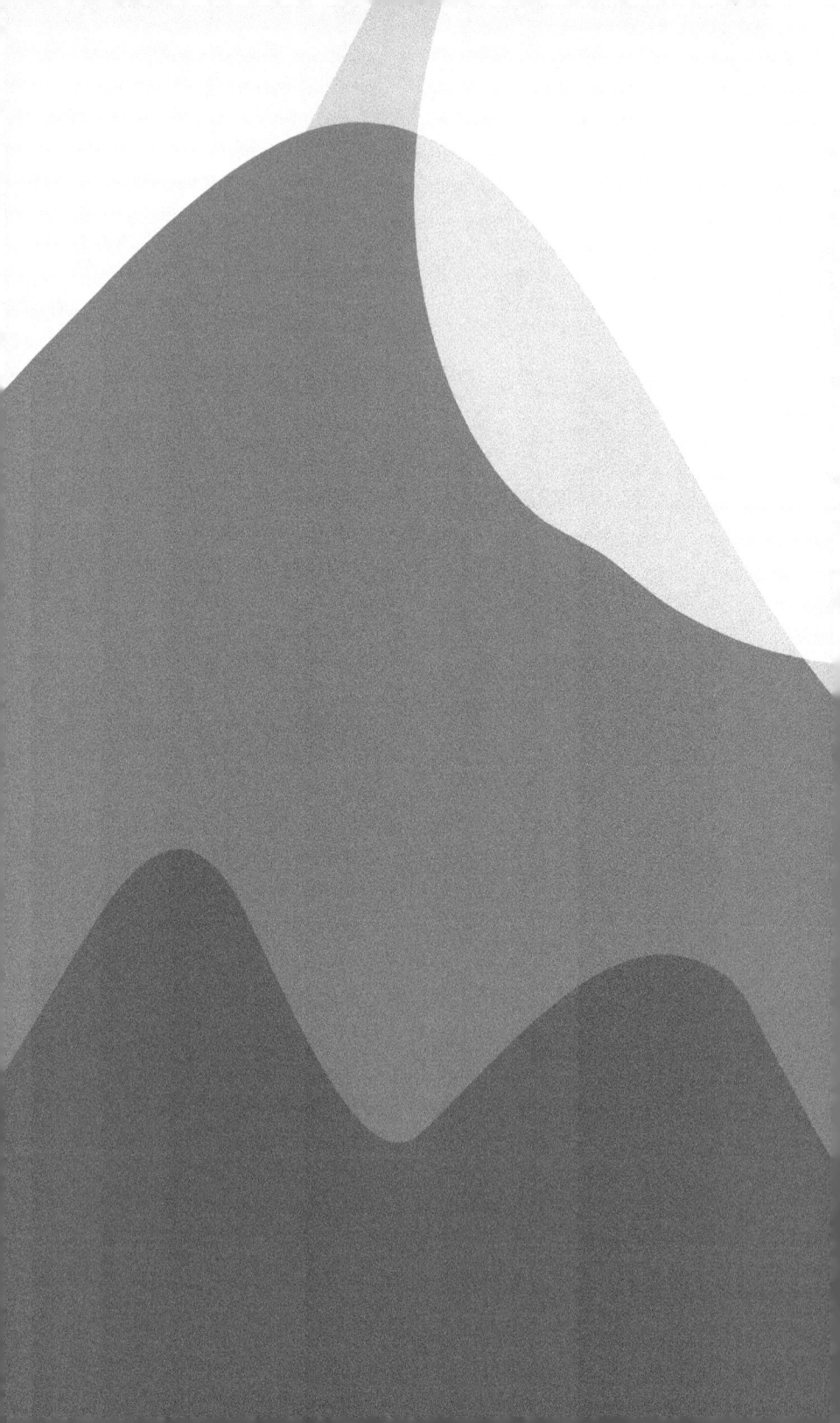

Time

There will never be a perfect time to say goodbye to someone you love. There will always be more hand holding to do and more hugs to share. How can anyone ever feel ready to say goodbye knowing their special someone is gone forever and won't be coming home again?

———————————

When I wrote this, my mom had just passed away and my heart was shattered in ways that felt beyond repair.

I write about loss and grief every single day, but after my mom died, I struggled to find the right words. Words that would somehow express the deep pain I felt as I stumbled around lost and numb.

Like so many of us do, I tried to find comfort in believing she had found peace and wasn't suffering anymore. I kept telling myself she wouldn't have wanted to linger on in pain or continue to live if she couldn't enjoy her life.

Rationally, I knew that to be true but it didn't make me feel better. It's hard to accept that my mom is gone forever. Losing her reminded me that it doesn't matter how old you are—you never really feel ready to let go of a parent.

I've been down this road many times before but losing my mom was a reminder that every loss is different. It doesn't matter how many people you lose in a lifetime, you never get good at grief, and every time you lose someone you love, it changes you a little bit more.

Regardless of how much you try to prepare, there's no perfect time to say goodbye to someone you love. Loss may be part of the human condition, but it's never easy, especially when the cold reality of permanence throws you into a brick wall.

Whether a loss is sudden or expected, the stamp of finality is painful and leaves a brand on your heart that's hard to accept. Honestly, my mom's absence still doesn't feel real and sometimes I find myself begging her to come back.

I desperately want to say good morning and hear the calm in my mother's voice. But the truth of knowing she won't answer my calls ever again breaks my heart open a little wider every time I reach for the phone.

The harsh reality of loss is no one is ever ready to say goodbye to someone they care about and love. It hurts so much to know they are truly gone and won't be coming back.

I'm a crier, and as I write this, tears are falling onto the page. I share this because I know you get it and carry the weight of grief in your own broken heart. There's a bond born out of loss and grief that ties all of us together.

People often say that your loved one will always be with you and while there's some comfort to be found in those words, I know it's not the same as having your loved one by your side.

I wasn't ready to say goodbye, but are any of us ever ready to let our loved ones go?

If you're reading this book, I'm sorry you know the deep pain of loss. I'm sorry you had to say goodbye to someone you love long before you were ready.

I know that holding your loved one in your heart and focusing on the love isn't the same, but it can help you to stay connected to them when trying to honor them and carry their legacy forward.

I still talk to my mom every day. I still write to her. I hug her picture and try to feel her presence in everything I do. I hope you can feel your loved one's presence too.

Please know that every word I write is written with love for all of our loved ones, for our grief, and for you. My heart stands in solidarity with your grieving heart and it always will.

It doesn't matter if it's been one day, one week, one year, or ten. There will be days when you struggle to believe the loss of your loved one is real, and sadly, no amount of wishing will ever bring them back.

––––––––––––––––

One of the most heartbreaking things about death is coming to the realization that there's nothing you can do to change what happened and regardless of how much time passes by, your loved one can't come back to you.

Accepting the finality of death is a difficult thing to do.

Waking up every day knowing your loved one is gone is like experiencing a thousand paper cuts to your heart over and over again. It doesn't matter how much time has passed, grief will continue to tap you on the shoulder and remind you that your loved one is still dead.

Yet there will be days when you wake up and still struggle to believe it's real. And if you're like me, you don't want to.

Being human means you will experience pain and grief. However, the gap between the ruthless days of unrelenting grief and the days when things quiet down will begin to stretch out, and the grief will no longer devour your every waking moment or haunt you in your dreams.

That doesn't mean you won't have days when you struggle, and even years later, there will be days when you miss them so much it stings and you don't want it to be true.

If you find yourself sad, crying, angry, or overwhelmed, let the feelings flow through you instead of pushing them deeper inside. Don't let them suffocate you. Feelings need to be released and expressed.

If you woke up today and found yourself struggling to believe your loved one is gone and nothing feels real, wrap yourself in a blanket of self-kindness and hold the memories against your heart. I see your grief and I'm sending you love.

The moment you know your beloved
is gone, time stands still. From that
moment on, life changes in dramatic
ways. There will be no more pictures
taken of them or memories made.
They will forever live in the past.

———————————

Honestly, it hurts to write this because I know how painful and dreadful the truth of loss can be. Time stands still when you lose someone you love and the future you were meant to share forever is just gone.

Oh, how that bitter truth hurts. It's a difficult part of life that no one should ever have to face.

The concept of time is cruel in the world of loss and grief.

One moment in time can change everything and regardless of how hard you try, there's no going back to how things were before a tragic loss tore through your life.

One of the most heartbreaking truths that comes with losing someone you love is the knowledge that there will be no more tomorrows to share or new memories to create.

There will be no more pictures taken, and the only choice you have is to look at pictures from the past. Loss literally stops time for your loved one and the ability to take new pictures and create new memories shockingly comes to an end.

There's no sugarcoating this side of loss and my heart hurts for you as you try to accept a truth that is cruel and hurts. What's being asked of you is too much for anyone to bear and yet here you are, being asked. Life can be so unfair.

The road of grief is long and it's hard to keep moving forward without your loved one by your side. But you move anyway because life expects you to and you need to keep moving to survive.

I know there will be no new pictures to put in a photo album or new memories to be made, but remember the love. Time can't take that love away and it's important to cherish the pictures you do have. Hold the memories and special times shared close in your heart.

Look at the pictures often and tell the heartwarming stories time and time again.

I know it's not the same and you will always yearn for more. I've never heard a griever say they spent too much time with someone they miss so much.

Loss has a way of reminding everyone of so many important things we forget and take for granted when life gets too busy. I know it won't change what's happened, but as you move forward, take the pictures, spend quality time with your loved ones, and build new memories every chance you get.

To say a picture is worth a thousand words takes on a whole new meaning when it comes to loss and grief.

One moment you were here and the next moment you were gone. And my life will never be the same again.

The death of a loved one is a loss that delivers an unforgettable punch strong enough to knock the wind right out of you.

Loss is a pain that soaks into every part of your being. A pain that's indescribable to people who don't personally know how awful losing a loved one is.

No one can prepare for that one moment in time. A moment that creates a gap between your life before and the life you're expected to live after losing someone you love. It's one moment in time when you can actually feel something burst and break inside of you. A moment that shatters and destroys you in ways you never dreamed possible.

It's a moment that can crush you physically, emotionally, and mentally. All at the same time.

When I received the news that there was a horrific boating accident and that my first husband's boat was potentially involved, I threw up on my bare feet in the grass and collapsed to the ground. I couldn't breathe and ended up in the ER shaking uncontrollably, numb, and in shock.

And when a friend of mine found her son unresponsive in his room from fentanyl poisoning, she screamed, begged, wailed, and kicked the wall.

I share this because I want you to remember there's no right or wrong way to react when one moment completely wipes out such an important part of your life. Do whatever it is you need to do to absorb the pain and shock. Don't fight any of it. Fall to the ground and wail. Throw up, scream, or kick the wall. Curl up in a ball and rock back and forth in silence. Whatever you feel in that awful moment, give yourself permission to be vulnerable and surrender to it.

The truth is, one horrific moment can alter your life in irrevocable ways and life won't ever be quite the same. And neither will you.

But human beings are incredibly resilient. It may not feel like it today, but you can and will survive. You will learn how to live life again even though it will look and feel different than it did before.

But it doesn't happen overnight. Adapting and adjusting to life after loss takes perseverance and time. It's not something you can rush through and some days will feel harder than others. Days when the pain of grief feels unbearable and it's hard to believe you will survive.

Don't quit. Life is a series of big and tiny moments, and while one moment can change everything, don't let it keep you from finding your way forward and enjoying the good moments in life again.

Lean on people who understand just how difficult grief can be. Find solidarity and comfort from those who are willing to sit in the uncomfortable and won't leave your side.

So much of the hard work of grief must be done alone but that doesn't mean you can't ask for help. Life may look different now, but you can choose to create a new life that allows you to live well and grieve well at the same time.

Please don't tell me it's been six weeks, twelve months, or five years. I'm painfully aware of every moment I'm desperately trying to live life without my loved one here.

Society has created a false narrative that the acceptable window for grieving is short and limited by an invisible timeline, as if crossing off days on a calendar will magically make grief disappear.

Let me be crystal clear. There are no limitations to how long someone can or should grieve. The belief that the first few weeks after a significant loss are the worst isn't always true.

Grief can't be restrained by a set of boundaries that don't actually exist. Much like love, grief is limitless and often meant to stay.

People who don't get it often say things like, "What do you mean you're still grieving? It's been six months!" or, "It's been over a year and it's time to get back to life and move on."

People say insensitive things, and unfortunately, so much of what's said places an unfair burden on the grieving to conform to unrealistic expectations. Sadly, many grievers question if they are doing something wrong.

This is unfair. Grief is a long process and for anyone grieving a huge loss, it's a process that may never completely come to an end. There's no hard stop when it comes to grieving and most people will grieve for their loved one until they take their last breath. Time doesn't magically fix grief; it's more about what you do with time while grieving.

Society needs to stop judging anyone who dares to grieve beyond the expected window of time. There's absolutely no truth to believing someone can grieve for too long. It's not about timelines; it's about your ability to eventually move forward in life even if you're still grieving.

And I promise grievers won't ever need to be reminded of how long it's been since they shared a final hug or were forced to say goodbye.

The grieving are painfully aware of every moment, day, and month without their loved one by their side.

People need to do a much better job supporting the grieving without judgment and paying attention to their words.

It doesn't matter how much time has passed. Your grief mattered the moment your world shattered and it matters now, regardless of how long it's been.

My heart will always stand with your grieving heart every day, every month, and every year.

Returning to work after a devastating loss can be difficult. People often have to go back to work long before they are ready and much too soon.

———————————

Contrary to popular belief, grief doesn't take time off or work from nine to five. Grief will travel with you to work and grief is rarely left at home.

Regardless of your job, grief tends to lurk in the shadows. And its presence is sometimes hard to ignore whether you're attending a meeting, checking emails, or sitting in the company break room.

Grief doesn't care if you have customers to help or deadlines to meet. And regardless of who's around, grief will sometimes demand to be heard.

It can be uncomfortable for managers, colleagues, and certainly grievers themselves. People don't always know what to do or say, and unfortunately, grievers often feel like they have to hide their grief away in a desk drawer and pretend like everything's under control when it's not.

In some ways, grief becomes a second full-time job. It can be difficult to find a balance between your responsibilities at home, doing your job, and navigating your grief.

The emotional and physical drain of grief can be distracting and debilitating. It's no wonder the grieving find themselves struggling to meet deadlines and lack the motivation and ability to perform at the same level as before.

Morale can take a hit and those who are grieving at work often feel isolated, misunderstood, irritable, and alone. How colleagues respond to a grieving coworker can make a huge difference when it comes to an employee transitioning back to work after a significant loss has rocked their world.

Sadly, too many companies fall short when it comes to offering support, resources, and time off for the grieving.

Whether it's due to a short bereavement leave or financial pressures, people are often forced to go back to work before they are ready.

Regardless of how much time you're able to take off, the transition back to work can be hard. On a side note, some grievers welcome going back to work, needing the distraction and a routine.

Give yourself plenty of compassion, don't be afraid to ask for help, and remember that struggling to concentrate is normal after loss.

You're grieving, and grief will show up whether you're at home or at work. I know it's a lot to manage and you deserve credit for trying. I'm proud of you.

There will come a time when you will say your last "I love you," share your last hug, or say your final goodbye. And when that time comes, it will hurt in the most unimaginable ways.

————————

After losing someone you love, the reality of "nothing lasts forever" becomes all too real.

We live life opening up our hearts and, with vulnerability, letting people in. We love, care deeply, and connect with others, and to be honest, experiencing a loving relationship is one of life's most precious gifts.

But loving and caring for others comes with a price. If you dare to love you will grieve and it's tough to grieve without feeling deep anguish and pain.

Love, loss, and grief are part of what it means to be human. Like it or not, every single person will eventually shake hands with grief.

Sadly, there will come a time when everyone will say the last goodbye and while you may not know in that moment, nothing can prepare you for how final everything will feel.

It's hard to understand the emptiness and pain that comes when you wake up and realize it was the last time for so many things. Things you would give anything to do with your loved one again.

It's true that most things won't last forever and we will all take our own final bow one day. But I do believe love lasts forever and in turn, so can the grief we carry.

I know it's lonely and I know it feels like so many people in your life don't understand your pain. And while that may be true, never forget all of the grievers who have walked the path before you and are ready to meet you right where you are.

It's hard to say your last goodbye to someone you love. It doesn't matter if it was a few weeks ago or if five years have passed. It still hurts and your grief will continue to exist because of love. If you love, you will grieve, but I believe it's better to love and grieve than to never know the beauty of love at all.

Most people dread the first year after losing a loved one. It's true there will be many firsts that are dreadful and incredibly hard. But the first year isn't a finish line to cross. There is no reward waiting for you and no promise that your sadness and grief will come to an end. You will continue to grieve after the first year, and sometimes the second and third years can be harder than the first.

Grief doesn't come with a well-thought-out plan or predetermined timeline. There's no final destination to reach, especially after a loved one dies. If the loss is deep and profound, grief can last forever.

Understandably, the first year after a loved one dies is incredibly hard. It's filled with endless firsts. Each of them feels like a gigantic hurdle to clear and the anticipation of most firsts comes with a sense of dread.

Whether it's a birthday, holiday, or the first anniversary of a loved one's death, the firsts without your beloved often come with deep yearning and sadness.

While you will get through the first year, surviving the firsts doesn't come with a guarantee that everything will magically get better or the grief you're holding in your heart will suddenly disappear.

Honestly, some people find the second or even the third year to be more challenging than the first.

Sometimes people are numb during the first year and find

themselves going through the motions in a state of shock. It can take a long time for reality to set in.

The first year can drag on or it can fly by as you're consumed with settling affairs, feeling overwhelmed, and simply trying to adapt to all that's changed. Every single first is undeniably hard, and it's important you take care of yourself as you grieve each and every one of them.

Keeping that in mind, grievers often find the second year to feel extra heavy and difficult to manage. The dust starts to settle and as the thick veil of fog begins to lift, reality hits like a sledgehammer delivering a crushing blow. The reality of forever sinks in and it becomes far too clear that this is your new life and your loved one isn't coming back.

Emotions will conflict with one another and as the sadness of the firsts spills over into the seconds and thirds, the finality of loss becomes all too tragic and real.

Whether you're experiencing the first, second, or third year, it will be hard. Adjusting to life without someone you deeply miss and love hurts beyond words.

Sometimes the anticipation of a first can be worse than the day itself, but whenever a moment, event, or day feels extra heavy, it's important to pay attention to what you need and to take care of yourself.

Grief will ebb and flow. It won't always be a constant and relentless stream of despair. You will get through the firsts, seconds, and thirds and while special days may always be hard, the grief will soften and fade into a gentle hum in the background instead of a loud banging in your heart.

I'm sending you extra encouragement as you dread some of the firsts, seconds, and thirds that lie ahead.

Time doesn't heal all wounds. Time helps you find ways to absorb the shock of losing someone you miss and love. Some of the wounds may never completely heal and perhaps not all wounds are meant to heal after loss shatters your heart.

———————————

To tell a griever after a devastating loss that time will heal all of their wounds is an outdated belief.

While it's true that time can heal and smooth out the rough edges of some wounds, there will also be those wounds that are so deep and painful they may not completely heal, regardless of how much time goes by.

There are people who come into our lives and leave meaningful, permanent footprints on our hearts. People who are so special, they change our lives in beautiful and unforgettable ways.

So to lose someone special is a cruel, heartbreaking reality that stirs everything up and wraps our lives in grief. And when the reality of loss hits, it's difficult to accept and hard to believe.

The footprint etched into your heart with love will remain but to live life without your loved one comes with a price no one should ever have to pay.

How does time heal something as brutal and devastating as that?

To lose a loved one leaves a hole that can't be filled. And while it's true you can replace many things in life, replacing someone you love isn't one of them.

Society will tell you enough time has passed. People will tell you to stand tall and that it's time to move on. You will hear words of advice you didn't ask for, and some of that advice will include hollow words that are trying to convince you everything's okay and you've grieved long enough.

Let's get real. There's no replacing a special person in your life. There's only holding on as tight as you can to the memories, pictures, and deep love shared. There's no replacing someone who made your life better. There's only honoring the life they lived as you learn how to transform and grow around your grief.

Time doesn't stop after a loss. Time keeps moving and there will be days when the concept of time is hard to understand. There will be days when it feels as if time has stood still and then there will be moments when it's hard to believe how much time has gone by.

Time doesn't heal all wounds. It's more about what you choose to do with time. However, time can help you to absorb the shock of losing someone you love, and over time you will learn to adapt and keep going regardless of how challenging it is.

And whether loss found its way into your life recently, or it happened years ago, both love and grief are now embedded into your beautiful soul.

Time takes on a whole new meaning after loss and the meaning is a reminder to take nothing for granted and to remember how short life is.

Grief doesn't care about time and time doesn't heal all wounds. And perhaps not all wounds are meant to completely heal. But if you can hold on, time will bring the gift of joy to your life again.

**Before you know it a year has passed
by and you are left to wonder,** *How
can that be? How can life have gone on
when my loved one is no longer here?*

The concept of time is always bittersweet when it comes to loss and grief.

The day that your entire world shifted and your loved one died can often feel like it was just yesterday. But then there are those moments when it feels like it's been forever since you last held their hand or heard their precious laugh.

Time will march on regardless of what's happened in your life. It doesn't care about the grief you now carry in your heart and soul.

Whether it feels like it's moving much too slow or flying by too fast, time doesn't stop for the living. It only stops for someone who dies.

When time stops for a loved one it's one of the most heartbreaking things to accept. It's devastating when reality punches you in the gut and you realize there will be no more dreams to follow, plans to make, or conversations to share with one another.

There will be no more hugs or new memories to build and that finality hurts in the most unthinkable ways.

Suddenly, time feels like the enemy. It can't be negotiated with or controlled. And before you know it, a year has passed by and you are left holding remnants of what was and wondering, *How is that even possible? How can life have gone on when my beloved is no longer here living their life by my side?*

Sometimes it's hard to make sense out of much of anything after a life-shattering loss. It is difficult to understand how time keeps ticking away and it's even harder to reconcile how life does go on. It can feel like time is pulling you farther and farther away from your loved one and the moment you were forced to say your last goodbye.

That's what happens in life and after loss. Life will pull you along with it whether you are grieving or not. And the truth is, life does go on.

I know it's hard to live one day without your loved one let alone one month or one year. Suddenly, forever feels like a really long time, and comprehending the brutal reality of what this all means is overwhelming.

There's no easy way to look time in the eye. It's normal to feel confused and even a little surprised as the days turn into weeks, months, and years. The passage of time is a heartrending reminder of how long it's been since you last heard your loved one's voice or saw their beautiful smile.

It's true you won't be able to slow the hands of time, but never forget that the love you and your beloved shared will never die. Time can't stop love and the gift of love is stronger than death.

I'm sorry you are hurting and I wish I could turn back the clock for all of us. Together we will continue to learn to live with loss and carry our grief one moment at a time.

It's Okay to Grieve

It's okay to smile and laugh after loss. It's okay to feel excited about something or get out and actually enjoy yourself again. It's okay to have days when you feel grateful and experience moments of joy. Your heart is big enough and resilient enough to hold both positive and negative emotions when grief becomes part of your life. And the truth is, human beings need a dose of joy once in a while to get through hard times and survive without guilt.

———————————

Guilt is common in grief and grievers tell me they feel guilty about so many things every day.

One of the biggest things the grieving seem to struggle with is feeling any kind of positive emotion after loss has left their lives in shambles.

People feel guilty if they dare to smile or laugh.

If they feel grateful for something in the middle of the mess.

If they have a good day and actually enjoy themselves.

If they look forward to something or feel excited again.

And the guilt feels extra heavy if moments of joy and happiness sprinkle their way into a griever's heart.

Sadly, grief can make people feel like they are doing something wrong if they laugh or smile. Somehow they believe they are forgetting their loved one or leaving their grief behind. It can feel like a betrayal to someone who has died.

To feel any type of positive emotion is alarming at first. Excitement, gratitude, or joy can feel confusing and conflict with all the heaviness that comes with loss and grief.

Sometimes the silent pull between positive and negative is exhausting. When positive emotions win the battle of tug-of-war, guilt and shame often step in.

I have felt guilty many times over the years. I pushed back against any type of good feelings and didn't think they deserved to walk alongside my grief.

I believed if I dared to laugh or feel happy, I was disrespecting my loved one and betraying my sadness and grief.

But here's the thing about loss and grief. It's a long and difficult journey, but you don't have to be chained to misery for the rest of your life. Grieving a heartbreaking loss doesn't mean you are doomed to a lifetime of anguish and despair.

Grieving doesn't mean you are destined for unimaginable suffering for the rest of your days, nor does it mean you are sentenced to a life of darkness and tears.

Grief is exhausting and you need a break from the heaviness and pain even if it's just for a short amount of time.

Human beings need both positive and negative emotions when grieving a significant loss. You need a little bit of light in your life to be able to navigate the darkness and find hope again.

You get to laugh and smile. You get to have moments of happiness and to feel grateful for the good that still remains. You get to have days when you feel less overwhelmed and peace brings much-needed calm.

You get to feel excited about what's happening in your life. You get to find the beauty and actually enjoy yourself again.

Your heart may be broken but it still has the capacity to hold all the same emotions it did before loss. Even though you've now made room for grief in your heart, remember that it's possible for joy to live next to it, side by side.

I know it can feel wrong when you laugh for the first time and I know the voice of guilt will be standing by to try to tell you it's not okay to smile or feel joy.

Don't listen. It's simply not true. It doesn't matter how much you laugh or cry. You will never forget your loved one or leave your grief behind. You may always carry grief with you and, while it may take time to get there, it's okay to live a happy and purposeful life again.

You may not be ready to hear any of this. If you're struggling to give yourself permission to smile and laugh, be patient and have faith that the smiles will return.

Grief is far bigger than one emotion and it doesn't always have to look like sadness and pain. Grief is a mixed bag full of mystery and you never know how it will show up from one day to the next.

Positive emotions are necessary when loss and grief become part of your life. There is nothing wrong with feeling happy or grateful. There is nothing wrong with laughing even though you feel sad, heartbroken, and lost.

Give yourself permission to grieve but also give yourself permission to find the good side of life again without guilt. It's okay. You deserve happiness and joy as much as anyone else.

The tears come without warning and sometimes at the most inconvenient of times. The grocery store. A yoga class. A party. During a work meeting or at school. Waiting for coffee in the Starbucks line. The holiday dinner table surrounded by family and friends. But that's okay. The tears are a reminder of all that's changed. A reminder of how much your loved one mattered and that they were here. Each and every tear that falls reminds you of how much you love them and how much they're missed. Every single day.

Here they come again. Uncontrollable tears, and every tear that falls seems to have a mind of its own. It doesn't matter what you are doing, where you are, or how many people are around.

And I don't know about you, but I'm okay with that.

Crying is a devoted companion to grief and whether it's a few tears or a full-blown sob, tears are a sacred testament to how much your loved one is missed.

Tears are part of being human and it takes courage to be vulnerable enough to break down and have a good cry.

The tears that fall are a gentle but compelling reminder of how much someone mattered in this life and that you miss sharing both the ordinary and extraordinary moments with them.

Tears are not a sign of weakness. In fact, whenever I witness a griever cry, I see tears blanketed by grace and bravery while trying to survive in a world that treats tears as childish.

Personally, I need to cry. I need to release all the bottled-up emotions trapped deep inside.

I've learned to let my tears fall and regardless of how inconvenient it might be or where I am, I give myself permission to cry. And so can you.

It might make others feel uncomfortable but after loss turns life upside down, you get to cry. As often as you need.

There's nothing wrong with tears. And I would be remiss if I didn't say it's also okay if you can't or don't cry.

Remember there's no perfect way to grieve. But if needed, please give yourself permission to cry. Tears are healthy, and you don't have to wipe them away so the rest of the world won't see your pain.

Loss and grief are hard and sometimes the only thing that brings even the smallest bit of relief is a good get-it-all-out kind of cry. Every single tear means something and you don't have to apologize.

I'm sorry you're hurting and I wish I could sit with you, tissue in hand, and give you a big hug.

Please don't tell me how strong I am. There's a big difference between being strong and somehow finding the strength to survive a loss that dismantled the life I worked so hard to build. Perhaps I appear to be strong on the outside but don't be fooled. On the inside, I feel broken and it's a struggle to carry this grief and pain. But I keep inching my way forward because I choose to keep going and live.

"You're so strong."

Sometimes, grievers don't like to be told how strong they are. To tell someone they are strong when they feel broken inside can feel like no one understands just how painful their loss is.

Loss rearranges life piece by piece and there are days when it can feel like you're hanging on by a thread as you buckle under the heavy weight of loss and grief.

Grievers often look okay on the outside because, unlike a broken arm gently reset and wrapped in a cast, a broken heart and the grief housed inside can't be seen. Sadly, people believe that if someone looks okay they must be doing better and moving on. Perhaps it's because that's what people need to believe because it's too hard to see a loved one in pain.

As unfair as it is, people often come to the wrong conclusions when it comes to loss and grief.

Appearances are tricky, and unfortunately, grief can't be seen from the outside. People will tell you how strong you are even though you may feel like you are crumbling and falling apart.

The grieving tend to struggle in silence. If society would just listen, they would understand that grievers don't always feel strong.

There's a big difference between feeling strong and having to dig deep and find the strength to carry on even when it feels impossible.

There's nothing wrong with finding courage and strength when grieving and sometimes strength does show up when you feel like you can't breathe through one more moment of grief.

But there will also be days when grief feels unbearable and you don't feel strong at all.

There will be days when it takes too much effort to cover up the pain and pretend to be strong just to please others. And what about the days you don't want to be strong?

Grievers need permission to be vulnerable and no one should ever have to act in ways that don't match how they really feel.

Even if you have days when you are defiant and strong, you don't have to be strong all the time. It's okay to stumble and fall apart. You get to sob in the shower or scream at the top of your lungs, "This really sucks!"

Grief will ebb and flow. Strength will rise and fall. You may feel strong one moment and crack the next.

But you don't have to be strong every day just to prove you're not weak. There's a difference between the two and I hope you remember it takes strength and courage to be vulnerable enough to love and grieve.

Let me be clear. There's absolutely
nothing wrong with you. You don't
have to justify your grief to anyone.
You're not crazy. You're not being
overly dramatic or a burden to anyone.
You're not too emotional. You're
not being too stoic or too strong.
You're not "fine" just because you
dared smile or laugh today. You're
not grieving for too long. You're a
beautiful human being grieving a
loss that changed you, your life, and
your world. No apologies needed.

There's nothing more frustrating than living in a world that some-how manages to make those of us who are grieving feel like we are doing something wrong.

I hear it from grievers every day. The doubt. The uncertainty. The shame. The fear. The guilt.

Recently, I worked with a client who lost her husband of thirty years. She was drowning in guilt because she believed she was cry-ing too much and grieving longer than she *should*.

Carol felt like she *should* be doing more to support her adult kids instead of grieving herself. And she felt guilty for not doing more to help her husband when he was dying and in pain.

The word *should* kept coming up, and the guilt was keeping her stuck in a place she no longer wanted to be.

Sadly, it's common for the grieving to struggle with guilt and shame. People feel like they have to hide their feelings from the rest of the world and often struggle to be honest with family and friends about how hard the journey of grief *really* is.

Fake smiles. Hidden tears. Doing too much too soon and trying to be the person others need them to be. Saying yes when they really want to say no.

It's miserable, exhausting, and unfair.

I get it and I've been there. I too have hidden my tears and pretended I was okay when the truth is, I was drowning in grief. I understand it somehow feels safer to play along with the unforgiving rules of society than admit to how much pain you are really in.

But I want you to remember one important truth today. Grief needs to be felt, witnessed, and expressed. It doesn't matter if you're an emotional griever or an intellectual one. It's necessary to find a safe space that allows you to express all your emotions or to take action instead of hiding them from everyone.

Unfortunately, society struggles with pain and grief. There is very little tolerance for the grieving process and grievers are often judged when they "feel too much, too little, or grieve for too long."

But here's the thing about grief. There are no time limits when it comes to grieving. There is no right or wrong way to grieve. Grief isn't meant to be silenced or confined. Grief is a natural and normal reaction to loss, and grievers should never be made to feel like they're doing something wrong. The grieving shouldn't have to justify their pain or grief to anyone.

If you take one thing away from these words, please know you're not unlike a million other grievers in the world. You're not overly dramatic or crazy. You're carrying a burden, but *you* are not a burden. You're not too emotional and if you don't cry, that's okay too.

You haven't reached the end of your grief journey just because you dared to laugh or actually enjoyed life today.

Don't buy into the false narratives of a society that doesn't always understand or support the pain of grief. You're an amazing human being grieving for someone or something you miss and love.

It doesn't matter what others think. They're not walking in your shoes and it's impossible for anyone to completely understand your loss and all you're personally going through.

Continue to meet your grief right where it needs you to be. Stop trying to please everyone else and don't be afraid to set boundaries when you're having a tough day or are feeling spread too thin. This isn't about everyone else. It's about you and your loss. This is about your grief journey and every step you take forward is brave. Every step you take counts.

Sitting in your loved one's chair,
wearing their favorite sweatshirt,
keeping their ashes on your nightstand,
or talking to them every chance
you get doesn't mean you're crazy
or grieving in unhealthy ways. It
means you're missing someone
you love deeply and it's love's
way of feeling close to them long
after they're physically gone.

———————————

The death of a loved one can make you feel like you've landed in a foreign country, desperately searching for anything that looks familiar. You feel completely disoriented and lost, and you don't speak this new language of grief. You yearn for the safety of home.

It's difficult to find things that bring you comfort in the early days, weeks, and months after loss. Everyone will grieve differently and when it comes to coping, you must find your own way.

Some people find great comfort in signs—to find a penny or feather, or to see a rainbow or eagle can be a gift that brings a sense of relief. Others visit their loved ones in the corridor of their dreams.

Comfort might mean sitting in your loved one's favorite chair, wrapping up in a favorite blanket, or wearing their sweatshirt while watching football on a crisp fall day.

Feeling close might mean keeping your loved one's ashes on your nightstand or wearing them in a pendant around your neck. It might be as simple as talking to them every time you go for a walk or before you go to bed at the end of a long day.

Regardless of what personally brings you comfort, there's nothing weird about it and there's nothing wrong with you.

However you choose to stay connected to your loved one is perfectly okay. To maintain and keep the bond of love strong even in separation is important and there are many different ways to honor your beloved after they die.

Personally, I find great comfort in all of these things and while it will never be the same as having my loved ones physically here, doing something to honor them gives me courage to keep going as I carry them with me. I'm wrapped up in my mom's favorite blanket as I write this and I hope you have found things that bring you comfort too.

And if nothing seems to help and you are struggling to function at all, it might be time to talk with someone and get the added support you need.

This is your grief journey and no one has the right to tell you how to move through your grief from one moment to the next. Find something that brings you comfort and give yourself permission to grieve. Regardless of what that something is, love will guide you, and I hope you feel the warm presence of your loved one today.

It's okay to be selfish when you're grieving and sometimes it's okay to be a crappy friend. Know your limits and remember, setting boundaries that honor your grief is the ultimate gift of self-compassion and self-love. It's having your own back in a way that no one else can.

———————————

Grievers often worry about what everyone else thinks. It's easy to get swept away in the current of trying to please everyone else instead of honoring your grief and living true to the person you've become.

If you're a self-diagnosed people pleaser like me, I want you to remember that it's okay to be a bit selfish when you're grieving. It's okay to stop trying so hard to do it all just because that's what the people in your life need and expect.

It's okay to say no, change your mind, or cancel plans.

It's okay to go to bed early, sleep in, or take a day off if you can.

It's okay to put things off. The dishes and laundry will wait for a day or two.

It's okay to retreat into yourself and not respond to every single text, email, and call that floods your inbox and phone today.

It's okay to talk about your loss, pain, and grief as much as you need to, even if people don't want to hear about it anymore.

It's okay to feel angry, sad, overwhelmed, frustrated, and exhausted.

And it's okay (and sometimes necessary) to laugh in between the tears.

Grief is hard and it can be difficult to know what you need. But you don't have to worry about everyone else all the time; it's okay to slow down and put yourself first once in a while.

It's okay to honor your pain and grief. To love yourself unconditionally with self-compassion as you try to figure out how to move forward and dig out from under the complexities of grief.

You're going through so much and sometimes you need to give yourself permission to be selfish even if it means giving yourself permission to be a crappy friend. The people who truly have your back and are willing to ride the waves of grief with you will understand.

Remember, there's no right or wrong way to do this thing called grief and it's important you allow yourself to feel and grieve in whatever way brings relief and comfort to you. No explanations needed and no questions asked.

You deserve a break and if being a little bit selfish gives you time to catch your breath, go for it without guilt and don't look back.

It's okay to grieve. It's okay if you're
having a really bad day. It's okay for
your heart to crack open and break.
Over and over again. It's okay that
you've changed. You don't have to
pretend or act like someone you're
not when parts of you no longer
exist. Loss does that. So give yourself
compassion and grace as you figure out
how to move forward in a world that
can feel so dark—one day at a time.

———————————

People tend to be incredibly hard on themselves, and sometimes
the expectations we put on ourselves are unrealistic and impossible
to meet.

Especially when it comes to grief.

Grief will wear you out. It's damn hard and depending on the
loss, grief is one of the most painful experiences life will ask you to
survive and endure.

Grief has no prejudice; it doesn't care who you are and it doesn't
care about geographical boundaries. It will find its way into the
lives of every single person on this planet. And it's not a mission
most people would ever ask for or choose to accept.

But it's a necessary one when you lose someone or something
you love.

I often think about how we talk to ourselves. Self-talk can be
negative, mean-spirited, and unforgiving as we try to navigate our
way through life. Especially when the universe asks too much of
us and loss sweeps through life with a wrecking ball and wipes so
much of what matters out.

It's so important to be kind to yourself when going through difficult times. To be patient and give yourself infinite grace. Tend to the broken parts of your heart and remember, it's okay to have days that feel unbearable and test you in unimaginable ways.

It's okay to have moments that challenge your will to show up and do the hard work grief asks of you.

There's no perfection to be found in grief. There's only finding a way to grieve that feels tolerable and manageable for you.

Unfortunately, there's a lot of pressure to "behave" in certain ways after loss. When people feel like they are grieving incorrectly, the pain can feel worse.

I know it's hard to focus on what isn't broken right now, but you deserve an abundance of kindness and compassion. And it starts with self-love.

Talk to yourself with kindness and stop beating yourself up. Write yourself a love letter filled with reminders that it's okay to stumble and fall. Give your heart permission to break. Post little reminders on your mirror, in your car, and throughout your home. Say these above affirmations over and over again.

You won't always feel this bad—and certainly not every day. You will have days when the sunshine melts your frozen heart and light finds its way back to you. You will have days when you smile and laugh again even if you sobbed in the shower earlier that morning.

Eventually, love and hard work will soak up some of your grief and dull the pain.

You're a warrior even when you don't feel like it. And if you remember just one thing today, remember it's okay to love yourself and it's okay to grieve.

To carry a smile and pretend like you're doing fine when the only thing you want to do is curl up in a cozy blanket and cry is exhausting. How can those who are grieving the loss of someone they love not feel tired and completely lost in a fog?

———————————

Grieving a devastating loss of any kind is difficult to say the least, and to find a way to balance everything that's thrown at you in the early days of grief can be incredibly hard.

There will be times when it's hard to get up, let alone find the courage to leave the safety of your home and venture out into a world that keeps on moving after your world has come to a stop.

It's exhausting trying to fit in or feel comfortable with people who effortlessly continue to live their lives as if nothing happened at all. And the truth is, as much as you want their world to slow down, they didn't just experience the painful disruption of a life-changing loss like you did.

Nonetheless, there's often a subtle but constant tap on grievers' shoulders from people asking them to do things that feel much too hard. The outside world desperately wants you to be okay and quickly move on from grieving. To paste a smile on your tear-stained face and pretend like everything's fine when it's not. To keep moving and fit back in because hiding your grief makes everyone else feel less threatened and more comfortable.

That's challenging for anyone grieving a difficult loss. It's exhausting to hold grief in and to give a daily award-winning performance that doesn't match what's truly going on inside of a griever's heart. It's a constant game of make-believe that asks people to pretend to be someone they're not.

But here's the thing. You grieve because you loved someone deeply and the grief you carry deserves to be felt, seen, and heard. Your tears deserve to fall and your heart gets to hurt.

You don't have to explain your pain or justify your grief. And if you're constantly feeling misunderstood or judged, it's time to let some people fall away and find a community who will love you and hold space for you *because* of your grief. A community that gets it and accepts you for who you are.

If you're grieving the loss of someone you love, tend to the wounds in your heart. Give yourself permission to sit inside the pain and cry as often as you need to. Let the pain wash through you as the tears fall.

Grief is hard but it's also a beautiful thing. To grieve means someone's life mattered. It often means you had the gift of loving someone and the gift of being loved. There's no better gift than that and that's what life is all about.

If you need to curl up in a cozy blanket today and cry, I hope you can find a safe space and the time to hide away from the world and let it all out. Nurture your bruised soul and aching heart. No performances required. You deserve that, so don't ever apologize for doing what you need to do and taking care of yourself.

Your grief belongs to you and you get to choose how to grieve. You get to feel angry, sad, and exhausted. You get to feel overwhelmed, lost, and afraid. You get to cry, kick, swear, and scream. You also get to have moments when laughter dries your tear-stained cheeks and the joy of the sun soaks up the darkness after the rain. And the truth is, you don't need permission to grieve from anyone but yourself.

It's easy to forget that we have the power of choice. And choice is a beautiful gift—most of the time.

With that being said, it's common for grievers to feel a loss of control because grieving isn't something most people would ever choose to do. But you will grieve after a devastating loss crashes into your life. And when life and death intersect, everything changes and it's difficult to accept something that forces its way in and becomes part of your life.

However, elements of choice do live inside your grief. You get to choose to grieve in whatever way feels right for you. People standing on the sidelines of your personal grief experience don't get to dictate how you should feel or grieve.

You get to feel anger, sadness, frustration, overwhelm, exhaustion, and fear. You get to feel uncertain, raw, and lost. Sometimes the pain is the only thing that makes sense when grief has left you feeling battered and life seems to be falling apart.

But you also get to experience joy and laugh when there are no more tears to cry. You get to feel moments of calm in the middle of the chaos. And thankfully, you get to rediscover beauty and hope when everything around you feels so cloudy.

You get to feel whatever is on your heart at any given moment in time and the truth is, grievers need to give themselves permission to feel both negative and positive emotions after loss.

This is your personal story, and sometimes choosing to feel all of your emotions is one of the only things that helps you to regain a sense of control. The pain that tends to accompany loss doesn't get to have the final word.

I know it feels as if there's no choice when it comes to loss, but you do get to choose how you grieve.

Bursts of grief happen at the most inconvenient and unexpected times whether you want them to or not. Give your grief the space it needs. You don't have to hide it even if it's in the middle of the produce aisle or checkout line in the grocery store.

It's difficult to predict when grief will take a stand and demand to be heard. Sometimes, grief will step out of the shadows at the most inconvenient time and in that moment, it can feel difficult to manage the sudden outburst of emotions depending on who you are with or where you are.

When grief ambushes people unexpectedly, the grieving often feel like they need to pull it together quickly or find the nearest exit dragging their grief out with them.

I get it. Suddenly finding yourself overcome with emotion in a public place can feel overwhelming, unsafe, or even embarrassing. Recently, tears found me in the middle of the grocery store. Shopping for a family gathering suddenly felt too painful knowing my mom wouldn't be there.

But I didn't leave even though I felt uncomfortable and didn't want people staring at me. I continued to shop with tears in my eyes knowing the moment would pass and the tears were falling because I was missing my mom.

Have you ever had an emotional meltdown in a place you didn't feel safe or comfortable? A place you felt compelled to hide your grief for fear of being judged?

While I want to stress that it's okay to grieve out loud regardless of where you are, I also know how uncomfortable it can be. Especially when you live in a world that doesn't always understand or support grief.

Your grief deserves to be honored even when it's awkward, and there's nothing wrong with grieving in public. But there will be times when it doesn't feel safe to be vulnerable and you need to find an exit and escape to a place you feel comfortable enough to grieve.

With that being said, sometimes you just need to let it all out regardless of where you are. And if you have a burst of grief when it's awkward and inconvenient, give yourself a pass. Even if it's at the dinner table, a party, or the store.

Grief doesn't always ask for permission but you can give yourself permission to grieve—regardless of what you're doing or where you are. It's a perfectly understandable, human thing to do.

There will be days when the only thing you do is grieve. And that's 100 percent okay.

We live in a world that doesn't always understand grief and sometimes people don't want to understand it. Sadly, the discomfort people often feel takes a huge toll on the grieving.

A false narrative has evolved over the years. A narrative that minimizes how painful grief really is. People expect the grieving to bounce right back into a normal life and soldier on.

Unfortunately, grievers often hide their grief or pretend that life is back to normal when normal no longer exists.

Tears are hidden behind fake smiles or quickly wiped away every time someone walks into the room. Crying is reserved for the privacy of the shower or the safety of a car and sacred grief stories are locked away never to be heard.

This helps no one. There are consequences that slowly emerge when grief goes unacknowledged or is hidden behind the curtains of toxic positivity.

Grief is meant to be felt and shared. It's meant to be experienced and not suppressed. There will be days when the only thing you need and want to do is *grieve*. That's normal. Regardless of how much time passes by, it's okay to take a grief day.

I know life is busy and I know life tends to pull you along whether you're grieving or not. There are endless lists of things that need to be done and it can be challenging to find time just for you, let alone time to tend to your grieving heart.

There's an epidemic of unspoken grief and like so many tough things in life, people struggle to talk about the ugly parts of grief.

People struggle to be present with all things that feel threatening or hard. Things no one wants to reveal or acknowledge.

But it's important and it's necessary. We need to change the conversation and normalize grief. Society needs to harness the big elephant everyone tries to ignore and lead it out into the spotlight.

Please be kind to yourself. Stop trying to please everyone else, and grant yourself the permission to do nothing else but grieve. You deserve those moments and so does your grief.

Your grief matters and you get to grieve. And if you're having one of those days when the only thing you can focus on is your grief, some of the other demands in life may need to take a back seat and wait.

I understand that you have responsibilities and there will always be things that stand in the way of taking the time you need. Do what you can when you can and remember, all grievers need moments when grief can stand on the center stage of their lives.

If you're having a day when your grief is suffocating you, I hope you can take time to breathe through it and just grieve. That's a perfectly acceptable thing to do.

People Don't
Get It

It can be hard to understand how everyone can walk around smiling and laughing. How can everyone get up, go to work, meet friends for dinner, and celebrate life as if everything is perfectly normal? Sometimes you might want to scream at the world. Doesn't anyone know what happened? Does anyone remember or care that your loved one is gone?

Life feels like it comes to a hard stop after a devastating loss. It can literally feel like the rest of the world keeps moving when your world becomes frozen in time.

It can feel like you're on a deserted island, stranded and alone. Left behind to sift through the wreckage of a life that changed in the most drastic of ways the day your loved one died.

My family and I were on vacation in Jamaica and I was pregnant at the time. I can still remember waking up and heading to the bathroom the day before we were due to fly home. My heart stopped the moment I saw a faint tinge of pink on the toilet paper. Fear crept in and as a tear rolled down my cheek, I pleaded with God to keep my baby safe. I couldn't go through another miscarriage.

As the day dragged painfully on, cramping set in. To make it worse, a huge storm blew in on the day we were set to leave and the streets flooded. I knew I needed to get back to see my doctor as quickly as possible.

Luckily, we were on the last flight out and as soon as we arrived,

I went to the doctor. I remember lying there staring at the ceiling while praying for a miracle that wouldn't come.

"I'm sorry; there's no heartbeat."

I felt a sudden stab to my heart, and the grief of losing yet another baby washed over me.

Both a D&C and a tubal ligation were scheduled for the next morning and even though it's been years, I still carry the painful memories of that loss with me. I was grieving the loss of my baby but I was also grieving the loss of my ability to have more children.

This miscarriage was one of many over the years, but it never gets easier. Every single baby I lost, regardless of how far along I was, was heartbreaking and cut deep.

I remember feeling abandoned and forgotten in my pain. People didn't talk about it—or at least not for very long. Everyone else quickly went back to normal while I lay grieving for the baby I would never get to meet or hold. I didn't understand how everyone else could move on so fast and return to life as if nothing had happened or changed.

I share this with you because any type of loss is terribly isolating, and watching the world keep moving is painfully hard to swallow and digest. Sometimes, it's tempting to scream out loud and remind the world of what happened, hoping everyone else will take your grief seriously and feel the pain of your loss too.

But they can't.

Even if people care, their world didn't change or come to a stop. It's not their responsibility or personal loss to bear and it's impossible for people to completely understand everything you're going through.

A heartbreaking loss of any kind can make you feel like you're no longer part of the world you're fighting so hard to live in. Somehow you no longer fit into the world in quite the same way. You exist in an altered state of being because pieces of your hopes and dreams are scattered about everywhere.

It's normal to struggle with relating to others after a significant loss. How can people be laughing or enjoying the day when your heart is crushed and you feel so sad?

Unfortunately, that's how life in the world of grief works. While your life is forever changed, everyone else goes back to their own lives.

But moving on isn't so easy for you. The world you once knew and even thrived in changed the moment your loved one died, and it's painful to observe the rest of the world acting as if nothing happened at all.

But your normal is gone. It's as if your life was blown apart in one painful moment, and the ground you once stood upon has crumbled, leaving a deep, empty hole.

It's not that you would wish your pain on anyone, but sometimes it's hard to witness others laughing, thriving, and enjoying the things you used to love. It's even normal to feel a bit envious as you struggle to fit into a world that has, in a sense, left you behind. To figure out a new way of living on your own.

I know it sounds hopeless, but please hear this: You will learn to navigate life again. You will uncover ways to find your place in the world again, even though it looks and feels so strange.

The world may never feel quite the same but remember you don't have to go through this completely alone. There are other people who are trying to fit back into the world after loss, just like you.

You don't have to stop sharing your story and the grief you now carry may travel with you wherever you go. Hold on tight to the memories and, regardless of what the rest of the world is doing, have faith that love and determination will hold you up as you find ways to return to life and figure out who you are.

There are no perfect words to take your pain away but please know you will always fit in with me. We are on this journey of loss together and even if you're struggling to find your place, it doesn't make you different from anyone. You're grieving. Coming back from your own personal and devastating loss is one of the hardest parts.

You can do this. I believe in you.

Just because someone is smiling, working, socializing, laughing, or functioning at all doesn't mean they are no longer grieving. It means they are trying to live and exist in a world that keeps moving even though something painful and terrible happened to them.

———————

One of the hardest lessons that comes with a heartbreaking loss is learning the truth that life doesn't stop even though your life has forever changed and very few things can go back to how they were before.

And while that's incredibly hard to reconcile, it's the brutal reality of how life works when loss turns life upside down.

Eventually, life pulls people along with it and for the grieving, it can be a time filled with conflicting emotions, including far too much guilt.

Society expects and needs people to get back to life as soon as possible. To return to a normal that no longer exists. Grief isn't something you move on from. You don't move on from loving and missing your loved ones. You learn to move forward and live life *while* missing and loving them.

But please plant this reminder deep in your grieving heart. Even though you may always carry grief with you, it's possible to live a fulfilling life again. When you feel ready, you can experience moments of peace, happiness, and joy. It's possible to smile, laugh, socialize, work, and function *while* carrying the deep pain of grief.

It's true that trip wires might lie in wait everywhere you go and there may always be things that try to derail you and knock you down. Things that pour salt into your wounds and tear them open again. But you will learn how to balance the good, the bad, and the ugly that continues to churn in and out of your life after heartbreak and loss.

I would encourage you to give yourself permission to feel the positive emotions and enjoy the good moments when they come your way. It's not a betrayal to your grief or your loved one. You don't have to feel guilty about it and the truth is, human beings need both positive and negative emotions to survive the difficult times in life.

You will learn to adapt to your different life. Thankfully, joy and grief can live together in harmony.

Society needs to remember that just because you're living your life and experiencing some of the good life has to offer again doesn't mean you're magically better or that your grieving is done. Nothing could be further from the truth.

Thankfully, the human heart is incredibly resilient. Even in the midst of pain, it's okay to laugh, smile, and find gratitude.

All of this may be hard to believe, and if you're not there yet, I understand. Don't give up. It's a long journey, and while you deserve to experience the good things in life again, the complex web of emotions you may be experiencing won't always make sense to you.

There's no right or wrong way to feel. Trust your instincts and listen to your heart. Go with what feels right for you in the moment and don't second guess any of it. You don't have to pretend to be happy when you're not. You don't have to feel guilty if you smile or laugh.

Life will be different in the most complicated of ways, but eventually the veil of darkness will lift and start to melt away.

Your grief deserves to be respected, acknowledged, and accepted—regardless of where you are and how you feel. And if that includes a good belly laugh, go for it and let go of the guilt.

Laughter is good for the soul and I highly recommend it once in a while.

Please stop expecting yourself to be the same person you were before loss destroyed some of the best parts of your life. You are not the same, and the person other people want you to be may not exist anymore.

A devastating loss of any kind brings about so much change it can literally feel like it destroys everything in its path.

Routines change. Dreams change. Plans change. Expectations change. Priorities change. Lifestyles change. The future changes.

People change.

And how could you not change? It's impossible to be the same exact person as you were before.

Loss tips everything upside down and scatters the pieces of your life carelessly into the wind. Nothing feels or looks quite the same and it can take a long time to feel grounded again.

Every part of this is normal after loss, yet we live in a world that doesn't seem to understand how much loss and grief disrupt life in the most unthinkable ways.

Family and friends often need or expect their loved one to go back to "normal." But that normal no longer exists and there's far too much pressure put on the griever to try to be the exact same person they were before their loss.

Typically, it's an expectation and need that can't be met. Loss changes people in ways that are hard to understand and can't always be explained.

Grievers sometimes struggle to recognize themselves and feel like a stranger in the world, their own home, and their own skin.

This can be incredibly unsettling and it's stressful when everyone around you needs and wants the old you back.

I don't know where you will land and I can't rescue you from the pain of grief. But I want you to stay the course and trust that with time, you can find pieces of your old self and the darkness will fade. The dense fog will lift and you will see glimpses of light peeking out from behind the clouds again.

With time, you will pick up the pieces and, one by one, it's possible to cobble yourself back together and settle into your new and different life. And instead of staying stuck in a state of limbo, you will become more comfortable with who you are as your journey of grief unfolds.

Some people will struggle to adapt to all the change, but the people who are meant to stay will love and accept you for who you are today.

People won't get it until they receive
a phone call in the middle of the
night, hold a loved one's hand as
they take their last breath, or find
themselves sitting in the front row of
a memorial service. People won't get
it until they wake up in the morning
with so much anxiety they can't
breathe, sob at a party because they
miss their loved one so much, or
have a deep ache in their soul that
never goes away. People won't get
it until grief shows up at their own
door—but I wouldn't wish the pain of
losing someone you love on anyone.

There are so many things that happen over the course of a lifetime.
Good things and bad. And some of those things are impossible to
truly understand until people experience them firsthand.

Whether it's having a baby, getting married, shattering a bone,
going through a divorce, or the death of a loved one, most won't
get it until it happens to them.

Keeping that in mind, there's a big difference in how the world
reacts to the joy of having a baby versus the pain of losing someone
you love. We live in a world that celebrates the happy occasions in
life but runs the opposite direction when life gets really hard and
grief shows up.

Society would never expect you to get over the excitement of
having a baby or the celebration of a wedding, so why do we live

in a world that expects people to get over a loved one's death? That makes no sense but it happens to grievers every day.

But perspectives change as soon as the heartbreak of loss pays a visit and turns someone's life upside down. Unfortunately, it takes personally losing someone or something you love to really understand just how hard the journey of grief *really* is.

It can be incredibly frustrating to feel like no one understands your pain. It's exasperating when people try to tell you it's been long enough and it's time to feel better and carry on.

The list is long when it comes to society and the many missteps taken in the land of loss and grief. So many ridiculous things are said to grievers. Things that are less than helpful and typically don't align with how a griever feels inside. People won't understand until they are forced to by experiencing their own loss.

It shouldn't be this way but it is.

It's my hope that we can continue to stand together in our grief and pain. To speak the truth and educate the world that it's okay to grieve. It's my hope that we can support one another and become more compassionate human beings because, like it or not, those who grieve get it and understand.

It's true that there are so many people who don't get it, but there are also so many people in the world who do. Loss happens all the time and eventually every person will come to know the reality of grief.

If you're struggling, connect with fellow grievers. They are carrying grief in their hearts just like you and it can be helpful to find someone to lean on and, in return, let them lean on you.

Please don't ask, "How are you?" The griever will most likely say, "I'm fine," and that might be a lie.

Grieving will sometimes make liars out of people. "How are you?" quickly becomes a loaded question: three dreaded words asked far too often. And while the words are not meant to cause harm, asking someone how they are can be problematic after a devastating loss.

It's a simple question and one that, in most cases, is asked with concern and love. But for the grieving, it can be a complicated one.

I appreciate knowing that people care enough to ask, but like so many fellow grievers, I struggle to know how to respond. Sometimes I want to say, "How do you think I'm doing? I'm grieving the death of someone I love" (or the loss of my marriage or the loss of my health—there are so many losses other than death).

With that being said, I often take the easy way out and simply say, "I'm fine," even when I'm not. How about you?

Sadly, it feels less complicated to tell people that you're fine and the truth is, the grieving often pretend because they don't want to make others feel uncomfortable or they don't want to feel judged.

And to feel the need to lie is unfair. People who are grieving shouldn't have to lie because it's easier for colleagues, family, and friends. People shouldn't have to pretend they are doing fine when they are anything but fine. The grieving shouldn't have to worry about making someone feel uncomfortable.

But grievers do—all the time.

I would like to believe that most people who ask genuinely care and are prepared to sit in the discomfort and hear the truth. But there are those who don't want to know the truth and in turn will walk away before a grieving soul can truly share how they really feel.

The journey of grief requires a great deal of balance and grace. It's complicated for the grieving and sometimes it's complicated for those who desperately want to support and help. I didn't always understand the importance or meaning of grace. But I've learned it's necessary to give ourselves and our loved ones grace during difficult times.

There are no perfect words, but perhaps it's best to not ask a question at all.

Don't put the responsibility on the griever. Just say, "I don't know what to say and I can't possibly know how you feel, but I can imagine how hard this is for you and I know your heart is hurting. I wish you didn't have to go through any of this and I'm here to listen or if you don't feel like talking, I will just sit with you for a while."

How does that land for you?

The truth is, there are no words or questions that will take the pain of grief away. But I know how much it helps to feel validated and understood.

It would be easier if no one had to lie when grieving. I hope you can find a safe space where you can be honest about how you really feel. A place where your grief has a voice and you can grieve out loud. You deserve that. We all do.

Broken hearts can't be seen from the outside but I can promise you if someone is grieving a significant loss, their heart is cracked wide open on the inside.

———————————

The truth is, the wounds of grief we all carry are invisible to the naked eye and we live in a world that doesn't always want to see the bruises of loss, a world that would rather focus on the shiny stuff in life and often tends to gloss over grief—even though it's part of life.

There's no right or wrong way to look, act, feel, or grieve, yet we live in a society that has far too many opinions and makes careless judgments based on false assumptions.

And from the outside looking in, society tends to believe people are doing well or getting better because grief can't visibly be seen.

Grief is far different than a physical illness or broken arm. There are no casts or bandages. There are no prescriptions to fill or take. There's no surgery or procedures to mend a broken heart.

Grief just is. And whether people can see it or not, the wounds of loss and the pain of grief are real.

It's so important to remember that just because someone looks fine on the outside doesn't mean they are fine on the inside. You can be standing right next to someone and have no clue they are hurting or what hell they are going through.

People are hurting all over the world, and after a heartbreaking loss, hearts are bound to crack wide open and split in two. But instead of offering love and support, people tend to step back and hide in the shadows in an attempt to sidestep anything that feels uncomfortable or is dripping with pain. It's as if grief is confined to a small space and blocked off by a no-trespassing sign.

But grief doesn't exist in a confined space nor does it want people to keep out or stay away. Grievers need people to cross that line and enter into their world of pain.

The journey of grief is a long and complicated one. Emotions will come and go but some of the emotional fallout from loss isn't recognized as grief and the world often assumes that if someone is functioning, laughing, or smiling, they must be over it and doing fine.

This couldn't be further from the truth and it's dangerous to make assumptions when it comes to grief.

If the loss is big enough, people often grieve for the rest of their lives, whether they look fine or not.

Your grief may be invisible to the outside world, especially if you're hiding it and pretending to be okay. But contrary to popular cultural beliefs, you get to grieve in the open. You don't have to get caught up in performing for a world that doesn't want to see or witness your pain.

You get to be a mess on the inside. You don't owe the world an explanation and whether people can see your broken heart or not, you should never have to justify how you look or feel to anyone.

You wouldn't pretend to be fine if you were physically sick or nursing a broken leg. You would tell the truth and ask for help along the way. Your broken heart deserves the same.

The pain and grief deeply planted inside your heart after a catastrophic loss doesn't end when the funeral is over and everyone goes home. The hard and exhausting work of grief is just beginning and it's long after the funeral when you need love, support, and compassion the most.

Wouldn't it be nice if all the people who called, sent flowers, mailed cards, stopped by, and dropped off food right after your loved one died would show up now? Even if a few weeks, months, or a year have passed by?

But some people have come to believe that the worst and most painful parts of grieving show up right after loss. Society thinks that pain and grief come to an end after the last card is read, the casseroles are gone, and the funeral or memorial service is done.

It's simply not true.

While the first few days after someone dies are drenched in sadness, shock, and pain, the hard work of grief is just beginning after the funeral is over and everyone goes back to their own homes and lives.

The week of the funeral is busy and, while devastated, grievers often feel distracted by everything they need to plan and do. There are phone calls to make, people stopping by, and arrangements to be made. It's a hectic time, really, and for a week or two, grievers feel surrounded by love and support.

Then, the funeral is over and everyone slowly disappears. Eventually, the last of the leftovers are heated up, the flowers are thrown away, and slowly, the phone calls, texts, and visits stop.

I wish it wasn't true but it's the way it works: The world will keep moving even though your world has changed in the most significant of ways. Suddenly, there's no more distraction and grievers find themselves alone and wandering through the halls of an empty house.

It can be disorienting at first and it's easy to feel trapped in a place that no longer looks familiar or feels like home.

The silence is deafening and regardless of how hard you try, there's no way to ignore the grief that now lives inside you. It's a long road, and when reality finally sets in, it's tough to distract yourself from the pain. The reality that you're forever changed and your loved one isn't coming back.

Society needs to do better when it comes to supporting the grieving. Society needs to stop minimizing the pain of grief and start recognizing that compassion is needed more than ever long after the funeral ends and everyone goes home.

Grief doesn't magically disappear but instead cements itself into your life and heart. Sure, grief shifts and the pain will fade, but even years later it can deliver a punch that knocks you off your feet.

Unfortunately, sympathy doesn't last as long as grief. And even though you may carry grief for the rest of your life, colleagues, friends, and family will quickly return to their own busy lives. Life goes on for them while your life has changed so drastically, it can feel like you're a stranger in your own life and house.

Slowly, the phone calls and texts fade away and people will reach out less and less. Some people will turn their backs on you and completely disappear. It's heartbreaking and while it's unrealistic to expect things to be exactly the same as they were in the first week or two, it would be nice if people would keep showing up regardless of how much time has passed.

An occasional phone call to check in, a heartfelt card, flowers just because, or coffee with a friend aren't too much to ask of anyone. Grievers need continued support.

I know it's lonely and I know how much it hurts to feel alone in the middle of the mess. And I know there are days when you need a safety net to catch you when you're trying so hard to hold it all together even though life is crumbling around you.

While words alone won't take your pain away, I hope some of these words provide a safety net of comfort, encouragement, and support today.

There are so many people who just don't get it. They don't understand how much courage and energy it takes to wake up every morning and grieve your way through another day. I see your grief and I'm proud of you for getting up every day. Regardless of how exhausting and painful it is, you manage to keep going and try again.

———————————

To say grief is exhausting is an understatement. Very few people seem to understand the toll grieving takes on you physically, mentally, and emotionally.

Grieving isn't for the faint of heart, especially after an unthinkable loss crushes your soul and breaks your spirit.

It takes a tremendous amount of courage to open the door of your heart and let grief in, and to keep getting up every morning to try to grieve your way through another day.

There's nothing simple about grief and yet there are countless stories of incredible resilience and determination to survive loss, trauma, and tragedy.

I know you're hurting terribly and I'm sorry there are people in the world who don't see your pain or understand how hard life feels for you right now. But people won't completely understand how much courage and energy it takes to survive a gut-wrenching loss until they personally become a member of this club that no one wants to join.

Grief has a hook in you that the outside world can't see, and sadly, it's common for a griever to feel completely alone.

Personally, I know how painful loss and grief are. And while no two losses are the same and everyone will grieve differently, fellow grievers do get it and have the hard-earned capacity to understand.

I will say it over and over again: I'm proud of you for getting up every morning and somehow finding a way to keep fighting your way back to life even in the face of loss and adversity.

I'm proud of you for surviving the heavy grief days and getting up every time you fall.

I'm proud of you for finding ways to keep your loved one's memory alive and staying connected to them even though they are no longer physically here.

I'm proud of you for the compassion and kindness you try to show others because you get it and don't want anyone else to feel completely alone.

I'm proud of you for staying the course even when you feel like giving up or giving in.

I'm proud of you for refusing to let loss and grief destroy you and choosing to forge ahead.

Because there will be days when it feels like the odds are stacked against you and no matter how hard you try to move forward in life, grief will sometimes pull you backward.

There will be moments when you're terrified to let go of the edge and fall without a parachute into whatever comes next. Moments when grief asks you to stay down but you get up anyway.

I know learning to live in a world that looks nothing like it did before is a big ask and it can feel like you're stepping onto a thin sheet of ice waiting for it to crack.

Eventually the ice will thicken and it will support the weight of your grief and pain. And if you have a day when everything feels too heavy and you fall through the cracks, it's understandable and okay.

Don't let fear paralyze you or keep you stuck. I hope the brave warrior in you will always remember the inspiring words of Mary Anne Radmacher: "Courage doesn't always roar. Sometimes courage is the small voice at the end of the day saying, 'I will try again tomorrow.'"

Keep doing your best, and even if society tries to tell you it's not good enough, hold your head high and don't apologize. They have no idea how amazing and brave you are. When the sun sets on another day, close your weary eyes knowing you did it. You survived another grief-filled day.

And that, my friend, is a big deal.

The insensitive words people say often make grievers feel dismissed and like no one understands their pain.

The platitudes. Empty and meaningless words that are shared far too often. Instead of bringing the comfort grievers desperately need, platitudes are useless and can quickly add another layer of grief and pain.

How many times have family members, colleagues, or friends said something to you that wasn't helpful or made you feel misunderstood or dismissed? How many times have things been said that didn't align with how you were really feeling inside?

Everything happens for a reason.

Your loved one is in a better place.

You will never be given more than you can handle.

Your loved one wouldn't want you to cry or be sad.

At least you can have another child or get married again.

Sound familiar?

The truth is, we live in a world that struggles with loss. Grief is thought of as an awful, messy emotion. One that's best to avoid.

And as sad as it is, people believe they are helping. Society believes some of these words will somehow make everything better and lessen the pain.

Grievers don't need advice on how to feel better and platitudes don't take away the pain of loss. Platitudes are dismissive statements that minimize the validity of grief. In short, platitudes can do more harm than good.

There are no easy solutions or silver linings to be found inside the pain. As Megan Devine so eloquently states in her book, *It's*

OK That You're Not OK, "Some things cannot be fixed; they can only be carried." Some losses cause pain and heartbreak that run so deep, people will always hurt in some way, and trying to tell a griever they will never be given more than they can handle is hard to swallow and challenging to believe.

Grievers learn to handle it because there's no other choice. People learn to manage their grief and address the pain because life keeps moving with or without them, regardless of how heartbreaking their loss is.

Most grievers I know don't want to hear their loved one is in a better place. Intellectually, this might be true if someone was suffering. But emotionally, telling someone their loved one is in a better place rarely softens the raw heartache of grief or takes their pain away.

The only thing grievers want is to have their loved one back and the only better place is right here. Living life. Sharing hopes and dreams. Together.

And while people may not want their loved ones to cry or be sad, the grieving are sad.

Grievers shouldn't have to justify their grief or apologize for their tears. Healthy grieving happens when people can be honest about their grief.

The problem doesn't lie with the grieving. The problem lies with a grief-illiterate world that struggles to embrace grief even though grief will impact everyone.

I know it's difficult to know what to say to someone who is carrying the pain of grief. We've all been there. Perhaps the best thing is to keep it simple. Sometimes less is more and to simply say, "I love you and I care," is enough.

I know words can feel hollow and meaningless and I'm sorry if anyone has said something that made you feel misunderstood and dismissed.

There are no perfect words but I can promise you I will never tell you everything happens for a reason or your loved one is in a better place. I will never tell you life will never give you more than you can handle and I certainly will never tell you to hide your sadness and tears.

This is your grief journey and everything you're feeling is valid. What you deserve is more love and support than you can handle. The pages in this book are platitude free and while words won't take your grief away, I hope you feel seen and understood.

"Please don't judge me for grieving a loss that turned my world upside down. Please be patient and respect my grief without looking at my story through your own lens. Everything feels overwhelming, and there are days I just can't do it all. Days I feel like I won't survive the pain. I'm exhausted and doing the best I can. My heart aches in ways that are hard to describe, and during this season of heartbreak, I need to do what feels right for me and not worry about what everyone else thinks or needs. I don't need you to fix me or cheer me up. What I need is love, understanding, and unconditional support."

———————

Every word I write comes from a deep place in my own heart. A heart that knows grief well. I share these words with you because I know how difficult the journey of grief really is.

I know how exhausting and lonely everything can feel when someone you love dies.

I want to scream as loud as I possibly can through the words I write with the hope that the outside world will hear how much they are needed when loss tears everything apart. I want to tell people to try to understand just how much your life has changed and that you're not the same person as before. To remind everyone of how heavy the weight of grief is to carry every day after losing someone or something so precious it hurts in ways that are impossible to explain.

I want to write a letter to your family and friends. To tell them to be patient and to please support you with unconditional compassion and love. To ask them to let go of unrealistic expectations and keep checking on you once in a while.

I know you're fighting a battle in the trenches of grief every single day. The battle is overwhelming, and fighting your way through the crowds of people who don't get it only adds to the pain.

I know you didn't ask for any of this and I know you're walking through a form of hell that's difficult to describe or name.

Please know my heart stands with you, and even though I have not had the gift of meeting you in person, I'm fighting in the trenches of grief alongside you. And while you must do the hard work of grieving alone, you're not completely alone.

Everyone needs a safe space to vent, share, and grieve. You need a place where you can be honest about your feelings and your pain. A place where you don't always have to hide behind forced smiles and pretend.

And if there are moments when you don't feel safe enough to be honest or you don't have the energy to stand up for your grief, it's okay.

The world can be an unforgiving place and to feel judged during one of the darkest times of your life is wrong. A time when it feels like all the stars in your soul have burned out and died.

I know the world doesn't always listen and I know there are far too many people who don't get it or understand. I'm truly sorry about that and I sincerely hope you can find a community of grieving hearts who will love you and embrace your grief.

This is your story and it's not a story to be told by anyone but you. You deserve love and understanding, not judgment, rejection, or unwanted advice.

I will continue to be a voice for you and all the grievers in this world. Grief was never meant to be silenced and your grief has the right to be heard.

Please don't tell me it's not that bad. For me, living life without my loved one really *is* that bad and I'm tired of pretending I'm fine when I'm not.

———————————

Oh, the ignorant things people say. Honestly, I'm blown away by the insensitive and dumb things people think and say to people who are grieving a life-altering loss.

I want to believe that most people share their thoughts with love and in some small way they are attempting to soothe the pain and help. But it doesn't change the fact that so much of what's said makes grievers feel dismissed.

It's true that the majority of people won't understand the deep and profound pain of grief until they themselves experience loss.

Nonetheless, to tell someone who is grieving for someone they love and miss every day "It's not that bad" is hurtful—and it's not okay.

There are losses that are so big and so heartbreaking, they hurt in ways that are difficult to comprehend. It really *is* that bad.

People often fail to register just how damaging words can be, and there's far too much judgment and shame in the world of grief.

I'm sorry if words have torn your broken heart open just a little more. It's not fair and I know senseless words can make you feel worse when you're going through one of the worst times of your life.

Honestly, the conversations in and around grief need to change and the people in your life who are less than supportive need to understand there's nothing more human than grief.

Having been through many difficult losses, I know it really is that bad for you, and I know how bleak facing a life without your loved one can be.

The truth is, one of the only things you can do with the huge boulder of grief sitting on top of your heart is learn to carry it with you as you rebuild your life.

I know that's not what you want to hear but please know it won't always be as heavy to carry as it is in the beginning weeks and months. Eventually, you will find ways to better manage your grief and when grief ambushes you, it won't be as intense or last as long.

Living life without your loved one will always hurt but it's possible to carve out a different life, and eventually, it becomes easier to focus on love more than pain.

Tend to your grieving heart and don't listen to what others think or expect. This is your journey and you get to have bad days.

On the days when you feel really bad, do something extra kind for yourself. Kindness won't take your grief away but it can make a difference and soothe the wounds you now carry.

There's a big difference between moving forward with grief and moving on from it. Society needs to understand the two are not the same.

We live and breathe in a society that continues to be uncomfortable with grief, and sadly, those who are grieving often feel pressured to get over their grief and move on.

But what so many people fail to understand is that grief isn't something you completely move on from. When grief shows up at your door, it typically becomes part of who you are, and it's tough to completely move on from something that you may always carry.

Moving on and moving forward are not the same. Yet, society consistently drops the ball when it comes to understanding how difficult it is to move on from a loss you will never forget. A loss that led you into the wilderness of grief. Regardless of how hard you try, there's no magical compass to help you find your way out.

Moving forward in life doesn't mean you've moved on, and relearning how to live in a world without your loved one is difficult. Stepping back into a life that's changed so much is unnerving, and even if you reach a place in the journey where grief and joy join hands, it doesn't mean you've completely moved on.

It means you've discovered a path forward with determination, bravery, and grit. It means you're slowly emerging out of the dense fog and creating a different life despite how much life has changed.

It means you've found a way to grow around your grief and the courage to keep moving when it would've been easier to give up.

With that being said, grief asks a lot of you and to walk a road covered in sorrow is no easy task.

There will be challenging days ahead and while it's possible to navigate through the vast and thick wilderness of loss, the grief you carry may accompany you every step of the way. Regardless of how much time goes by, it's challenging to completely move on from it or leave it behind.

Human beings have the capacity to survive. Even after a tragic loss tears everything down, people find ways to move forward and rebuild.

There's a knowing that comes with the raw and painful experience of loss. People who have walked the well-traveled road of grief will get it and understand.

Don't give in to anyone who doesn't understand your pain or coerces you to get over it and move on. Life has asked far too much of you and while it's possible to slowly move toward new beginnings, grief may continue to travel with you. And that's okay.

If moving forward and rebuilding feels impossible right now, give yourself compassion even when others can't. Breathe deeply through the difficult moments and try to keep moving one small, admirable step at a time.

Please don't tell me to get over it. The "it" people refer to has become part of who you are, and just like you will love your person forever, you may grieve for them forever.

There's a lot of injustice in the world but when it comes to loss and grief, it's so unfair when the outside world lacks compassion and tells the grieving it's time to get over it.

It's ridiculous to tell someone who is fighting every day to bear the unbearable pain of loss to suck it up, get over it, and carry on.

Grief isn't something that suddenly goes away. People don't just get over a loss that ripped their soul wide open.

The death of a loved one (and other losses too) is heartrending. The grief that follows is often heavy, complicated, and packed with pain. It's a life-changing experience that's extremely personal, and if the loss is significant enough, it's rare anyone will grieve for a short period of time and completely get over it.

The scars of loss form quickly and even though things won't always feel as harsh or intense as they do in the beginning, grief tends to stay. People need to find the courage to carry grief forward as they crawl their way back to life and figure out how to survive in a world that doesn't always understand their pain.

The "it" society casually refers to isn't something the grieving get over. The "it" is a sacred part of the before that will always be housed in a griever's heart.

And just like love will always remain, so does grief. Remember, you grieve because you love. You grieve because someone or something made a difference in your life.

If you're grieving, you don't have to get over it. Don't bend to the pressures thrown at you from a society that's so obsessed with finding happiness that it comes at the expense of feeling any pain.

And when you're willing and ready to clear a path and move forward in life, stay true to your heart and cling to the love. Your loss and grief matter because of that love and the "it" will stay with you forever because it's supposed to.

And there's nothing more human than that.

You're not the same person you were before. Your life has been split in two. One side of your life is all about pretending everything's okay, and the other side is screaming in silence from the indescribable pain of loss. It's really hard to climb out of the rubble and rebuild in a world that no longer makes sense or feels safe to you. And the truth is, there may be days when you find yourself struggling, when you feel you're not okay.

We live in a world that can be unforgiving when it comes to grief and the window for grieving out loud is far too short.

As unfair as it is, life keeps chugging along and the pain of grief can leave you feeling untethered from the world, lost in the middle of a sea of grief.

Sadly, the world doesn't always show up in the way grievers need. There are few lifeboats sent out to rescue grievers when the storms of loss hit.

Life after loss feels unsettling and it's no wonder people feel so afraid and alone. There's an element of desperation, a need to be saved from the pain and uncertainty as grief unfolds. A desperate clinging to anything that looks vaguely familiar and will keep you above the murky waters of loss so you don't sink into a world of hopelessness and grief.

It's really hard. And I mean hard in ways that are difficult to comprehend until you've personally descended into the underbelly of loss and grief.

Nothing's simple and life can feel like a huge mess filled with no direction and far too many loose ends.

It's like living two lives at the exact same time, and frankly, the fatigue and exhaustion can feel impossible to manage in the middle of the complexities of loss and grief.

In the early months after loss, part of you is trying to exist while attempting to meet the demands of daily life. You might be acting like everything is fine while the other part of you is hurting terribly and it's a struggle just to open your eyes in the morning and drag yourself to the shower or get dressed.

The grieving often suffer in silence and instead of screaming and letting it all out, they hide the pain and sadness away until there's a safe place to be vulnerable enough to truly grieve.

It's like walking a tightrope and trying to balance everything without a safety net to catch you when you fall. And my heart hurts for anyone who's constantly being pulled in two completely different directions day in and day out.

I know how hard it is to hide your pain so no one else will know. And as wrong as it is, the ability to be honest and truly grieve is often reserved for stolen moments when you're alone.

There's a component of loneliness that cuts right through the pain. How nice would it be to live in a world that unconditionally holds space for your unbridled grief?

But the truth is, we live in a world that struggles with sadness and people will try to encourage you to smile, look at the bright side, and fix your grief.

It's hard to rebuild a life that feels as if it's been destroyed at the hands of loss. It's hard to climb out of the rubble when you feel so defeated and you're forced to live two different lives while simultaneously trying to protect your heart and please the outside world.

I can't change the world we live in, but I want to encourage you to find people you trust and a place you feel safe enough to grieve out loud. With time, you will rise above the rubble and rebuild a different life. A life of acceptance where you don't have to pretend to be someone you're not.

And you can be a guiding light for someone else who is feeling lost and alone. Sometimes it's when we can help others that we can better help ourselves.

There will be losses that are deemed unworthy of grief by a society that clearly doesn't understand that no two losses are the same. However, every loss is valid and deserves to be grieved.

_____

Grief is always complicated but there are some losses that seem to come with an extra layer of complexity. Losses that are often judged and misunderstood.

Some losses are stigmatized and lead to disenfranchised grief when the outside world doesn't acknowledge the loss and deems it unworthy of grief.

Grief is lonely regardless of the loss, but if you're carrying the pain of what society thinks of as an unacceptable loss, the isolation can feel unbearable.

Have you ever felt like you had to defend your grief?

I know I have, and sadly, it happens all the time.

I've had people tell me they felt alienated after losing an ex-husband or ex-wife. For some it was the death of a friend, a partner, or suffering the pain of a miscarriage. Others have shared they are grieving for someone they had an estranged relationship with or someone they didn't know.

Millions of people around the world grieved when Princess Diana died. I will never forget the heartbreak I felt when I heard about her death. Even though I never met her, I loved and respected her, and the grief I felt was real.

When my first husband died it was a complicated time that left me feeling isolated, judged, and alone. We were divorced when a tragic boating accident claimed his life as well as the lives of four other young men.

Even though we were no longer married, I still cared deeply about him and in some ways felt like a grieving widow who wasn't allowed to grieve. To make it even more complicated, I had remarried just one month before.

But here's the thing about loss and grief. It doesn't have to make sense to anyone else and it's impossible for the outside world to understand the relationship, the attachment, or to know the depth of your love, grief, or pain. Divorce happens for many reasons and when two people let each other go, it doesn't always mean the love is completely gone nor does marrying someone else cancel out every emotion and feeling. It's possible to love more than one person in a lifetime.

In full transparency, there were so many reasons for the grief I carried all those years ago. He was the father of my two oldest daughters, who were just six and eight at the time, and he was still one of my best friends. We talked almost every day and continued to do things together with our kids. I was grieving for the father of my children and my heart was breaking for my girls. I was grieving for a man I had known since high school. A man I would always care for and worry about. I was grieving for all of the things he would never experience and would miss out on in life. I was grieving because he would never see his daughters grow up or walk them down the aisle. I was grieving for all the men who died that holiday weekend and for their families and friends. It didn't matter that he was my ex; I was grieving, in part, because of love.

Honestly, I was devastated and the grief was so heavy I struggled to function. But I needed to tend to my kids' grief and, as the rest of the world quickly reminded me, I had a new life now. I shouldn't be grieving him. I needed to get over it and move on.

To be fair, I had a few people who continued to support and

show up for me, and I'm eternally grateful for them. But most of the time, I felt invalidated and judged, like I had to hide my pain and grief. There was no place for my grief to go, and it sucked the life and joy right out of me. I found myself comparing my loss to others' and some days, I felt guilty for grieving at all.

Looking back, I know my grief mattered and regardless of a piece of paper, my grief deserved to be expressed, validated, and heard.

The truth is, you can grieve for someone you've known for forty years and you can grieve for someone you barely know or have never met. You can grieve for an ex or someone you had a falling-out with many years ago.

You can grieve for a beloved pet, a colleague, or someone who bullied you. You can grieve for your health, the loss of a job, or your home.

You can grieve for a child you carried and never held. You can grieve for the child you always wanted and will never have.

Miscarriage, infertility, exes, estranged relationships, addiction, overdose, suicide, abortion, pet loss, stigmatized diseases like AIDS, health, divorce, the loss of an extended family member or friend, adoption, losing a job or home—all of these things and so many more often fall into the category of disenfranchised grief. It's unfair for any loss to be put into a category that forces grief underground.

There are no rules when it comes to grieving, and grief shouldn't be harnessed or contained. There's no room for judgment, comparison, or competition when it comes to loss and grief.

But disenfranchised grief happens and it can smother someone's ability to grieve when the outside world doesn't acknowledge the loss or consider it to be worthy of grief. It forces people to grieve in silence and can lead to added pain.

Let me be clear: Every loss is valid and worthy of grief. My grief isn't more important than anyone else's grief. It's just unique and personal to me. And your grief is unique and personal to you.

It's not wrong to grieve for someone or something you cared about and loved. The who, what, when, where, why, or how doesn't matter. Please don't listen to the outside world. Don't let anyone judge you or minimize your loss. Your grief matters just as much as anyone else's; don't ever feel ashamed for feeling the deep pain of any loss that breaks your heart.

It can be hard to name our grief when it feels unacceptable to others or complicated in some way. But it's important to be able to talk about your loss so you're not holding everything inside. If you ignore your grief for too long, the dam will break and it will spill out in unhealthy ways.

I promise your loss matters and you deserve to have others bear witness to your grief and pain. Regardless of the situation, you deserve love, comfort, and support. Don't settle for less. Remember, you don't ever have to justify your grief to anyone.

The Many
Faces of Grief

A day in the life of grieving:
Wake up feeling exhausted. Think
about your loved one. Feel sad. Have
a cup of coffee. Walk around the
house feeling lost and numb. Cry in
the shower. Go to work. Hide behind a
fake smile. Feel sad and overwhelmed.
Need to cry but don't. Tell people
you're fine when you're not. Drive
home exhausted and cry. Do laundry.
Talk on the phone. Feel grateful. Make
dinner. Nurse a throbbing headache.
Struggle to believe this is real. Wash
dishes and cry. Watch a show. Relax
and laugh. Feel lonely and go to bed.
Miss your loved one and feel empty.
Sob into the pillow. Pray for sleep.
Wake up feeling like you didn't sleep
at all. Pull yourself out of bed and try
to survive another day all over again.

A day in the life of grieving will look different for everyone, but regardless of where you are in your personal journey, a day in the life after loss can feel like an exhausting and challenging grind.

Did you ever see the movie *Groundhog Day*, starring Bill Murray? The movie is based on a self-centered weatherman named Phil who finds himself in a time loop on Groundhog Day, and the day keeps repeating itself until he gets it right. As frustrating as it is for Phil, the movie is also an undeniable call for hope.

While grief isn't about "getting it right," it can feel like you're trapped in a time loop and stuck on repeat. One day rolls into the next, and the exhaustion of grief can take a huge toll. Some days feel like a thankless job of survival, and the truth is, there will be days when it feels easier to quit and be done.

Even though you may want to hit the snooze button and stay in bed, life drags you along. Days can be filled with so many different emotions, all at the same time.

There will be moments when you feel fine and the next minute you're fighting back the tears. There will be times when you feel worse, better, and then worse again.

Life doesn't slow down for grief, and for most grievers, life feels overwhelming and the list of things to do never ends.

There are kids to take care of. Bills to pay. Shopping, cleaning, and going to work. There are meals to prepare, grass to mow, and dishes to wash. Perhaps you have been invited to a party or there's a soccer game to attend.

Whatever fills up your schedule, it's tiring when grief is running alongside you day after day. It is a Groundhog Day of sorts and it can feel like things will never get better or change.

And to make things worse, people often feel like they have to hide their grief and keep up when the only thing they want to do is close the curtains, climb back into the safety of their bed, and have a good cry.

I get it. I know and understand how overwhelming and exhausting some days are. And while I can't possibly understand exactly how you feel, I understand how upsetting it is to wake up and be stuck in the same loop time and time again.

Grief isn't a one-size-fits-all experience and everyone will grieve in their own personal way. You will have your own grief itinerary and even that will change depending on how you're feeling or what's going on that day.

It may not feel like it, but we are all in this together and while you must manage most of your days alone, there are people who understand and want to be there for you.

Life can feel like a daily grind and one that seems to be stuck on repeat from one day to the next. I know it's hard, but you do have the power to break free of that endless time loop that can keep you feeling stuck. I hope today will bring you happiness and, like the movie, I hope you find the courage to keep on. Eventually, you will find a renewed sense of hope.

Grief can feel like a wild and untamed beast. One minute you're treading water and doing okay. The next minute a powerful wave hits and you're pulled back under the surface of life where pain and anxiety live. When it's a struggle to catch your breath, we all need a life raft to help us stay afloat.

———————————

Grief is one of the messiest experiences you will encounter in life. It's constantly changing shape and asks people to change with it and color outside the lines.

I wish I could tell you that grief is predictable, but to put it bluntly, it can be a wild and untamed beast.

Grief is disorienting and it will make its presence known when you least expect it and at the most unsuitable and awkward times.

Thankfully, you will have moments or even days when everything feels manageable and you actually see light at the end of this very dark tunnel. Days you start to believe you will be okay. It's a welcome and much-needed sense of relief. And then, boom. You're pulled back out to choppy, deep water and it's a challenge to find your way back to the safety of shore.

Suddenly, the world tilts and shifts. The pain of loss rears its ugly head and the reality of grief crushes your soul all over again.

One minute you're having a wonderful time laughing and the next minute you're lying on the floor in a puddle of tears. One moment you're enjoying dinner with friends and the next minute you're curled up on the couch watching *Eat, Pray, Love* for the tenth time, sobbing into a bowl of ice cream or Lucky Charms.

That's how grief goes. Regardless of how hard you work to establish a sense of stability, grief will continue to show up and kick the legs out from under your chair, reminding you it's still there.

I won't pretend the journey of grief is easy, and frankly, the early days, weeks, and months following a significant loss can feel so unpredictable and intense, it's hard to manage it, let alone feel secure.

When a wave of grief hits without warning, it's easy to feel defeated and left to wonder if you will ever be okay.

There will be moments when the pain is undeniable and it's difficult to imagine living the rest of your life without your loved one by your side. There will be moments when you feel like you won't survive the day.

I understand.

When I lost my best friend in a devastating accident, I truly didn't think I would survive. I believed I was destined to live a life in darkness without hope or the ability to find the beauty or good in life again. But with time, I slowly emerged out of the darkness and light found its way back into my life. I learned it was possible to move forward when you find courage and choose to return to life alongside your grief. It was possible to find glimmers of joy, smile, and laugh again. To find purpose and meaning even though grief had become a permanent tattoo on my heart.

There were plenty of setbacks and I still have moments of sadness and grief. I will never tell you it's easy and I won't glaze over how devastating and difficult the journey of loss is. It's damn hard. But grief doesn't have to be an infinite cycle of darkness and pain. You can choose to move forward and beyond the darkness even if you have to crawl through the mud to get there.

Time will keep moving and eventually a week, month, and year will pass by. Sometimes it will be hard to believe just how much time has come and gone.

I know how deep the pain of grief runs after losing someone

you love. Even years later, grief can erupt out of nowhere and while it may not feel as intense or last as long, the waves of grief can still knock you down.

Don't give up. Eventually this beast called grief will become more tolerable and tame. And on the days you're fighting to swim back to the surface and tread water in this new and unfamiliar life, let the words in this book bring you comfort and throw you a life raft whenever you need one.

The early days, weeks, and months can be brutal after a devastating loss. You may sleep too much or struggle to sleep at all. You will struggle to focus at work or work harder than ever before, hoping to distract yourself from the pain. The simplest of daily tasks may feel hard to complete as you try to juggle emotions that are running wildly out of control. And sometimes you might find yourself laughing one minute and crying the next for no reason at all.
That's grief.

Grief doesn't always make sense. You need to give yourself grace as you figure out how to live life again when everything you try to do and all of the emotions you're carrying inside somehow feel all wrong.

The bigger the loss, the bigger the grief. A devastating loss will change you and your view of the world.

Everything will feel in disarray and it can be a huge challenge to step back into a life that doesn't look or feel anything like it did before.

The early days, weeks, months, and even the first year or two will challenge you in the most unexpected ways, and finding your way back to living life in a world that doesn't miss a beat can feel like an impossible ask for anyone grieving a gut-wrenching loss.

It's common for grievers to struggle with transitioning back to daily life after loss tips everything upside down.

People often find themselves sleeping too much or lying in bed for hours battling insomnia, struggling to sleep at all. Going back to work too soon creates anxiety and some people struggle to focus and get anything done. Others work extra hours hoping to find a distraction from the relentless pain of loss.

Even the simplest of daily tasks can feel overwhelming yet the demands of life keep piling up and life can quickly become unmanageable.

Sometimes you feel too much and then there are days you're too numb to feel anything at all. It's a wild ride. When grief collides with the demands of life, it can feel like you're sinking to the bottom of a hopeless pit with no lifeline to pull you back out.

It's normal to feel sad, angry, and irritable. And yes, sometimes you might feel like you're a shitty family member, colleague, or friend.

One minute you might find yourself laughing hysterically only to burst into tears the next.

Don't fret. It's all normal. Please cut yourself huge amounts of slack and stop beating yourself up. You're grieving and it can take a long time to find a rhythm in life again.

Regardless of what you may have been told, you won't grieve for a few days and then get back to normal or move on. Grief isn't a reality TV show or a Hallmark movie where everyone lives happily ever after because the movie is over.

There are no stages to check off a list when it comes to grieving, and the journey of grief isn't linear. Grief is messy, unpredictable, and dances all over the place, making no sense at all.

It's true that grief can be difficult to control and predict from one day to the next but you will slowly come to understand your own grief and learn how to best carry it forward.

No two losses are ever the same but I promise you're not the only one feeling out of sorts and struggling to survive a loss that ripped your life apart. There are and will always be pioneers of grief who broke ground before you and understand your pain.

Regardless of whether your grief makes sense to you today, you're not doing anything wrong. I hope you can let go of the guilt and replace it with grace on the days when grief feels like a tsunami of overwhelm and despair.

Take it one moment at a time, my friend. If you're running on empty and the only thing you're capable of doing today is surviving, let that be enough.

Grief is unpredictable. It's anger.
It's pain. Grief is love. It's yearning.
It's sobbing in the rain. Grief is
overwhelming. It's guilt. It's feeling
shame. Grief is messy. It's regret. It's
smiling when you say their name. Grief
is exhausting. It's heavy. It's bold and
loud. Grief is soft. It's laughter. It's
comforting. Grief is bittersweet. It's
a quiet hush. It's lonely even in the
middle of a crowd. Grief is human. It
shifts and changes from one day to the
next. Grief may last forever. It's part
of who you are now and who you will
become. Grief is a beautiful testament.
It honors your loved one's memory.
Grief is here for a reason. Grief isn't
the enemy. So let your grief be a
gentle guide and don't push it away.
Every loss matters so give yourself
grace and permission to grieve.

———————————

I have been writing poetry since I was a young girl. For me, writing
is the calm in the middle of the storm. It's therapeutic when life is
falling apart and it's a way to release the pain and breathe.

You don't have to be a writer to find the benefits in writing.
It can be a poem, writing a letter to a loved one, or sharing your
deepest thoughts in a journal every day.

You don't have to show your words to anyone or you can share
them with the world.

I write because it's a way to express the complex feelings and emotions that ride on the wings of grief. I write from a place of love and I write from the heart for you.

I write with the hope that some of these words will be companions that provide a soothing and relatable balm to your wounds and broken heart. I write with the hope that they provide an emotional lifeline when you feel isolated and alone.

Loss will clip your wings when you really want to fly, and I'm sorry you have come to know the deep pain that comes with loss and grief.

Grief is so many things. It all matters, and you don't have to hide what it means to be human anymore. In the end, never forget that most of the grief you carry is because of love, and you can learn to fly again.

Anger often gets a bad rap and is unacceptable in the eyes of the world, but the truth is, anger is sometimes a necessary emotion when it comes to grief. It's normal to feel angry after loss blows your future hopes and dreams apart.

When I ask people what grief looks like, the most common answer is sadness, and while sadness is a big part of the grief experience, grief is so much more than feeling sad.

The journey of grief is wrapped up in a complex web of emotions and it's normal to experience anger after a life-changing loss tears pieces of your life to shreds. Yet people don't connect anger to grief. If anger flares, society deems it to be an unacceptable emotion, one to control and avoid.

Anger has a bad reputation. It makes people feel uncomfortable and the grieving tend to suppress their anger and hide it away. Anger is an emotion that can feel confrontational and people often push their anger aside.

But when it comes to loss and grief, anger is sometimes necessary and it can be a healthy reaction when things feel threatening, hurtful, and unjust.

Anger is a frequent guest at the table of grief and it's important that we, as a society and as fellow grievers, remember it's okay to feel angry after loss.

Anger is a form of self-preservation and a way to protect one's heart. It's a way for people to reclaim their power instead of feeling out of control and helpless. And when anger flares, it may be a front concealing other feelings, including guilt and fear.

It's impossible to turn back time, change the outcomes, or fix what's happened—and that's difficult to accept.

But that's the reality of loss, and when grieving, anger doesn't have to be the bad guy. Anger can be useful. Anger can address so many of the unfair and painful things that happen in life. It can rise up and stand guard when you feel threatened and you're too weary to fight back. Anger can help you to feel like you're taking action and doing something to meet your grief head-on.

If you're struggling, remember that it's absolutely okay to feel and express your anger. It doesn't work to suppress it for too long, and if you don't deal with your anger, it will swallow you up and eventually come out.

Anger isn't necessarily good or bad. It shouldn't be judged but rather accepted as a legitimate emotion that pulls up alongside your grief. Anger can serve a purpose as long as you don't let it consume you or impact your life or relationships in unhealthy ways.

It starts with awareness and recognition. Name your anger, feel it, and learn to accept that anger is a necessary part of grieving. Don't run away from it. You can't outrun grief or anger; it will always be one step ahead of you.

If you're feeling angry today, stomp around, swear, punch a pillow, go for a run, scream out loud, have an ugly cry, throw a temper tantrum, or have a meltdown. Own your anger, feel it, and honor it. Just like grief, your anger is there for a reason and that reason is called loss.

Grief fog is real after loss breaks your heart and rewires your brain. It can be difficult to remember all of the things you're supposed to do from one moment to the next. So please be patient and try to be understanding with yourself if you forget to call or text someone back. Forgive yourself if you cancel last-minute or feel like you haven't heard a single word someone has said. Don't judge yourself if you forget to eat or need a day to lie around in bed. Go easy on yourself and let it go if you're too tired, emotional, angry, or sad. Don't worry if your grief makes other people uncomfortable or if you're not the same person you were before. You may not know who you are right now or what you want or need. Honestly, you're doing the best you can, and you need that to be enough.

_____

Grief is a journey that's hard to explain to anyone who hasn't personally experienced the pain of loss. Grief rarely follows a straight path and there will be days when it feels like the life you're trying to live is a knotted-up mess.

That's the hard reality of grief, and as much as people will try to minimize your pain, there's nothing sweet or sparkly when it comes to how complicated grief can be or how much it hurts.

Loss changes people and some of the ways grief manifests are difficult to understand.

It can feel like you're floating through the middle of a thick fog, and without a road map to guide you, it's easy to feel disoriented and lost.

The fog I'm speaking of seems to engulf your mind, body, and heart, making it difficult to move and keeping you stuck.

I remember feeling so disoriented and exhausted after my dad died. After years of battling alcoholism, his body gave out and he couldn't fight what had become a lifelong demon anymore. On top of that, I had a newborn and spent my maternity leave at the hospital with my dad, feeling helpless, frustrated, and alone. It was a traumatic experience on so many different levels.

There were days he didn't know who I was and it was painful to watch him deteriorate physically and mentally as he slowly slipped away. And when he died, I felt both gutted and relieved.

Following his death, I struggled with PTSD. Everything felt scattered in my brain. I felt guilt, anger, and sadness, and the struggle to concentrate was real. I had my baby and a toddler to worry about, but there were moments when I felt lost in a fog and regardless of how many times I showered, I couldn't wash away the smell of my dad's hospital room.

The simplest of tasks overwhelmed me and, other than taking care of my kids, I couldn't see beyond the fog. It was, to say the least, a really challenging and painful time.

Have you been struggling with poor concentration or feeling forgetful and detached?

Are you more absent-minded than usual or having a hard time focusing, listening, or following through on things?

Rest assured there's nothing wrong with you. Grief brain happens all the time and while it can be unsettling or feel like you're losing your mind, it's normal after loss shakes everything up. It's normal to feel like your emotions and thoughts are a scrambled mess.

The fog that seems to coat your brain can linger for a long time after loss. If nothing makes sense or you feel confused, please know it's normal and with time it will begin to lift.

All bets are off when you are tasked with facing the daily grind of life while carrying so much pain and grief.

Everything that was once familiar tends to shift and change. And the smallest of tasks can feel impossibly hard. It can feel as if grief has robbed you of your sense of direction and clarity.

Don't beat yourself up if you find yourself forgetting things or need to dial back and rest. You don't have to figure everything out right now.

Give yourself license to let go of self-imposed expectations that are tough to meet from one moment to the next. It's normal for moments to slip through your fingers and to forget big and small things.

There are no quick fixes when it comes to the fog of grief but there are a few things you can try.

Make lists or use sticky notes to help you remember all the things you need to do. Write in a journal. Let go of unrealistic expectations and know your limitations on those extra hard days. Set a timer. Reduce distractions in any way you can. Use a calendar, whether written or on your phone. Meditate to relax, or get outside for fresh air to clear your head. Stay hydrated and rest.

If you're struggling with grief brain, be patient and have faith that eventually the fog will begin to clear and clarity will return. Stop worrying so much about the unrealistic demands of a world whose ground didn't give way and collapse like yours did.

You're grieving and there's nothing more understandable and normal than that. Be who you need to be right now and stop being so hard on yourself. And if you feel like you are suffering from trauma or PTSD, it might be helpful to talk to a therapist.

You don't have to know the answers today. The answers will come. Grief may always be part of the journey, but eventually, it will blend into your life and not feel so obnoxious and loud.

Please remember you're enough and it's absolutely 100 percent okay to grieve. Go easy on yourself every time the fog of grief takes over your heart, body, and brain. It will pass.

After a loved one dies, the anticipation, anxiety, and fear of losing someone else is terrifying. As the possibility of another loss lingers in the corners of your mind, the what-ifs feel far too real.

Fear and anxiety are common emotions that go hand in hand after a devastating loss. It's impossible to ignore the cluster of conflicting emotions that tug at your heart and flood your mind when grief comes knocking at the door.

Every day will look and feel different. Grief is unpredictable and some of the ways grief shows up won't always match your beliefs of what grief should look like. Some of the feelings you encounter won't make sense.

People forget how complicated grief can be. And it's easy to forget that grief can look, feel, and sound a million different ways.

There's a lack of recognition when it comes to the many emotions that make an appearance after a soul-crushing loss. People expect to feel sadness but it can feel confusing when anxiety and fear creep in.

And so many emotions experienced with grief are deemed unacceptable even though they are natural, normal, and often necessary after the heartbreak of loss.

Honestly, we need both negative and positive emotions. All emotions play an important role in life and every emotion should be acknowledged and processed.

You can oscillate back and forth between positive and negative emotions many times a day. And as short as positive thoughts might be, they are important and can provide a window of respite from the heaviness of loss and grief.

But herein lies the challenge. Sadly, people don't always recognize that so many of their emotions are deeply connected to their grief and the pain of loss.

Fear and anxiety are two powerful emotions grievers often experience after losing someone or something they love. Loss can leave people feeling vulnerable and fragile. It's a reminder that life doesn't come with promises or guarantees. For anyone.

Losing a loved one turns the volume of fear and anxiety way up and it's normal to fear losing someone else. It's easy to sit on the edge of anxiety ruminating and waiting for the other shoe to drop.

Before loss upends life, people tend to get comfortable with what can be a false sense of security. They look at the world through a rose-colored lens and, right or wrong, believe bad things only happen to other people.

But bad, awful things do happen to people every single day and if you're reading this book, I'm guessing something awful has happened to you. I'm guessing the color has temporarily drained right out of your life and you've been forced to look at the world through a different, grief-stained lens.

I'm guessing you have a front row seat to the heartbreak of loss. To live life personally knowing that no one is immune to the pain of grief is scary, and it makes sense that you're struggling to feel safe and secure.

It makes sense when anxiety and fear burrow deeply inside of your mind, and it's normal to worry something bad could happen again. Your comfort zone has been crushed by the trauma of loss, and it can be a challenge to feel safe in this new and different world.

To accept the finality of death, knowing we have no control over it, is difficult. It's easy to feel powerless and, if left unchecked, anxiety can lead to a full-blown panic attack.

Having lost a couple of special people in my life to tragic accidents, I struggle with anxiety and fear. I dread when my phone rings in the middle of the night or when friends and family are driving on Minnesota roads in the middle of winter.

I freeze up and struggle to breathe when I'm riding as a passenger in a car or on a boat. My brain often comes up with all kinds of scenarios and images that leave me feeling terrified of accidents or losing someone else. While irrational, the fear holds me hostage sometimes.

When fear and anxiety are present, it can feel like you're constantly waiting for the next catastrophe to happen. Suddenly, the world can feel like an unsafe place.

You may find yourself trying to control everything around you, and instinctually, you may be extra vigilant and protective regardless of what you're doing, where you are, or who you're with.

But here's the problem with constantly living on the edge of fear and waiting for something bad to happen. Anxiety and fear are exhausting and both can suck the peace and joy right out of you. If you're so busy worrying, it's easy to miss all of the beautiful things you deserve to experience and see.

All of the worrying, fear, and anxiety in the world won't necessarily protect you from more loss and pain. The truth is, terrible things do happen. Loss happens every single day and while many of our fears never come to light, there's no guarantee, regardless of how vigilant you are.

You may always carry grief in your heart, and believe me when I say I understand the grip of anxiety and fear after losing someone you love and care about.

It takes self-awareness, work, and commitment to calm your anxiety and fears. Honor the parts of you that feel terrified and anxious. Face your fears but don't let them paralyze you and keep you from living your life.

If you're feeling anxious, remember to breathe. Take deep, intentional breaths through your nose and exhale your worry and fears through your mouth.

Step away and try to do something that brings you comfort. Something that might relax you or bring you a sense of peace. Think about a memory that makes you happy. Try writing out your feelings or taking a long walk. And if anxiety and fear are controlling you, talk to someone.

Listen to what your mind and body are trying to tell you. I'm sending love and calming thoughts your way.

Losing someone you love is tragic, and it hurts in ways that are hard to explain or comprehend. It's emotionally draining to constantly yearn for someone or something while knowing all of the yearning in the world won't bring them back. Life can suddenly feel like a game of survival and to live life after a deep and profound loss is one of the hardest things anyone will ever have to do. Yet you do it one small, painful step at a time.

Anyone who knows the heartbreaking pain of losing a loved one knows the deep yearning I'm talking about.

It's incredibly difficult and there will be days when it's hard not to reflect on what was and what could have been. The wishing, yearning, and longing for something that just can't be is, to put it bluntly, gut-wrenching.

Grief isn't something you master or become good at and no amount of toxic positivity or cheering up will make everything all better or take the yearning away. And as hard as it is, grievers must learn to live and hopefully thrive inside of a life that won't ever look or feel quite the same.

Yearning is part of the grief experience. It houses the ache of knowing you can't put things back together in the same way as before. Yearning is normal and sometimes the ache is so powerful it can feel like it's pulling your heart right out of your chest.

If you're anything like me, I'm guessing you have moments

when you would do anything to go back in time and experience the good parts of your life all over again.

Yearning is human and it's a common response born out of a devastating loss. It can stir up the pain and heartbreak over and over again as you yearn for something or someone that won't be coming back. Some days it's scary and it can feel like a sad, tragic movie that has a beginning but never ends.

You will always yearn for what was and will never be, but the intensity of yearning will eventually quiet. It won't always feel like it's devouring you. I know it's hard to believe, but you're more resilient than you realize and you will find ways to move forward as you learn to coexist with grief.

The grief and yearning don't completely stop and maybe they're not meant to. How could you not grieve and yearn for someone who meant so much to you?

Your heart and brain will slowly learn to process all the changes that come with a devastating loss, and eventually you will find ways to adapt. You can learn to manage the sorrow and you won't always feel so disheveled and lost.

Don't put undue pressure on yourself to rush toward an end to your grief that may not exist for you. If the loss left a huge hole in your heart, there may be no final destination to reach and, even years later, the presence of grief often remains.

If the ache of yearning has cast a dark shadow in your heart, it's my hope you will find the smallest reflections of light as your day unfolds. While nostalgia can feel bittersweet, let yourself remember and soak up the warmth of love and your beautiful memories.

A life-changing loss can feel as if
it's sucked all the oxygen from your
universe, and honestly, grief is so
much more than feeling sad. Grief will,
at times, inhabit every part of your
being and if you have days when you
need to lose your shit, go for it. You
don't have to justify it to anyone.

———————————

When I ask people what they think grief looks like, the number one answer is crying and sadness.

There's no doubt that one of the most common and intense emotions in grief is a deep and profound sadness. And there will be moments when it feels like the sadness will never subside or go away.

While grievers tend to feel sad for a very long time, there are so many other ways grief shows up and makes itself known. Grief isn't just an emotional experience. Grief impacts people physically, spiritually, and mentally too.

Grief is unruly and complex. It's easy to feel trapped in a web of feelings that conflict with one another and don't always play nice in the sandbox.

Grief will look different for everyone and the list of how grief can manifest is long.

Grief looks like distraction, staying too busy, or not feeling motivated at all.

Grief looks like shutting down and sleeping too much or not enough.

Grief looks like an excruciating headache, a full-blown panic attack, or feeling so depressed it's hard to get out of bed.

Grief looks like overwhelm, anger, envy, and guilt.

Grief looks like forgetfulness, loneliness, fear, and feeling lost in a fog.

Grief looks like happiness, gratitude, joy, and peace.

Grief looks like going out to celebrate and laughing with friends.

Grief looks like splashing in mud puddles and dancing in the rain.

Grief doesn't look like just one thing and it's possible to experience all of these or none of them at all. Regardless of how grief shows up for you, every day can look different and it's hard to predict how you will feel.

There may be moments when there's so much going on inside of you, you don't recognize who you are and it's easy to feel a lack of control. I know it can be unsettling but please know that it's all normal and there's nothing wrong with you.

Grief may not be easy to control, but that doesn't mean it has to control you. With that being said, grief does need space to breathe and to be expressed.

And as hard as one might try to hide it or repress it, grief will force its way to the surface. If ignored, it might come out in less than desirable ways.

Grief isn't a singular emotion. Everyone grieves in their own unique way and how grief shows up for you may be completely different than it is for a fellow griever standing right next to you.

That's normal and what matters the most is that you are able to recognize that so much of what you're feeling is acceptable and may be connected to your grief. Self-awareness and tending to your grieving heart can help you to begin the process of healing and moving forward.

The road of grief is long and it's confusing sometimes. Be patient as you sort through the messiness of your emotions and, at all costs, be kind to yourself.

It's a lot to manage, and honestly, if you need to lose your shit once in a while, go for it.

You still can't believe your loved one is gone. No matter how much time goes by, you may not want to believe it's real.

One of the most painful and difficult things about losing a loved one is actually believing they are gone.

It can take a long time to come to terms with the fact that someone who was such an important part of your life is never coming back to you.

Ouch. Even writing these words stings. The reality of loss sucks and to adapt to life without your loved one in it is inconceivable.

Everything feels out of balance and there will be times when you feel like you're trying to walk uphill with a five-hundred-pound boulder strapped to your back. No matter how far you climb, you can't reach the top and get to the other side.

It's hard to come to terms with the fact your loved one is actually gone. Rationally, you know it's real, but emotionally, it takes time for the heart to catch up and there will be moments when their absence feels surreal.

I've experienced this a lot in the past year. I will look at my mom's picture or reach for the phone to call her and for a brief moment, it doesn't register that she's truly gone.

I still struggle to believe it's real.

It would be easier if we could all just pretend nothing happened and try to forget the pain. But you won't ever forget. The void in your heart expands and contracts with each painful day and, as hard as it is, no amount of pretending will change what happened or bring them back.

Forever is a really long time, and suddenly, your loved one is just gone. It's tough to accept and it's natural to struggle with disbelief.

It's normal for the grieving to wake up and momentarily forget their loved one has actually died as they reach for the phone or turn over to say good morning in what's now an empty bed.

I can't change what's happened and I can't take your grief away but it's my hope that as you relearn how to exist in the world, you will also find ways to keep your loved one close to your heart while keeping their memory front and center in your life.

It can feel difficult to stay connected when the only thing you want is to have your loved one sitting right next to you. But remember, love never dies.

It's important to acknowledge your grief and to practice the best in self-care when grief is weighing heavily on your mind, body, and heart.

The reality of loss and all that's drastically changed will continue to challenge you as you struggle to adapt to a different life. A life you didn't ask for but now have to live.

I know it's hard to believe; most people don't want to believe it's true. The journey of grief is difficult but tomorrow is another day of new possibilities and the chance to rediscover hope.

And as hard as it is, it's essential to face and accept the truth regardless of how painful it is. My heart stands with yours and even when you're struggling to believe it's real, I will never tell you how you "should" be feeling or how to grieve.

Grief is incredibly lonely and it's easy to feel invisible and alone even when you're standing in the middle of a crowded room.

———————————

Sadly, grievers are some of the loneliest people in the world and the isolation some people experience is heartbreaking.

Loneliness becomes part of the journey when grief settles into the folds of your heart. And even if you have a supportive network of family and friends, it can still feel lonely. Because it is.

No one knows the depth of your pain better than you and no one can grieve for you. And while others may think they understand exactly how you feel, they can't.

Having said that, there are also things that people do and say (or don't do and say) that add additional layers to the loneliness so many grievers already feel.

Unfortunately, people rarely bring up the loss or acknowledge the grief resting heavily in a griever's heart. Grievers feel invisible and sometimes feel alone even when standing in the middle of a crowded room.

It happens all the time.

And while grievers may try to talk about their loss with family and friends, their words often fall on deaf ears and so many responses from loved ones lack genuine compassion and interest.

I would like to believe that people mean well and some genuinely want to help. But it doesn't change the fact that grievers often feel empty and alone.

Oh, how I wish I could erase your pain, but as much as I want to, I can't completely fill the deep hole in your heart. Even the most comforting of words won't take your loneliness away and the truth is, no matter how much people love and care about you, it will never be enough. Your loved one will still be gone.

However, my heart stands with yours and I understand the deep and relentless ache of loneliness that becomes a steadfast companion inside of your grief.

I understand the feelings of isolation and literally how awful it is to feel invisible even when people are around.

It hurts, especially when you feel like no one gets it or cares enough to truly listen without judgment or giving unfiltered advice.

I know your heart breaks a little more every time you feel unseen, especially when you're going through one of the most painful experiences of your life. Also, it can be a time overrun with conflicting emotions. Sometimes you want people around and sometimes you crave silence and need to be alone. To sit in solitude and sink into the depths of your pain without having to explain or talk to anyone.

However you're feeling in the moment, trust your heart.

Grief *is* lonely and in some ways it will always feel lonely. But there are communities of grievers who understand the unquenchable loneliness that can seep into the cracks of your mind, heart, and home. Communities who will welcome you and your grief with open arms offering validation, sympathy, and love.

In a perfect world, you will find comfort and acceptance with your closest family members and friends, but sometimes it's a stranger or casual acquaintance that becomes your biggest supporter when you're feeling miserable.

Even on your loneliest days and when you feel like you might shrink and completely disappear, I hope the pages in this book will remind you that you're not completely alone.

I'm sending you love and light with every single word I write.

The truth is, you will never stop missing them. How could you stop missing a person you love more than anything in the world? There's no forgetting, replacing, or completely filling the void that now sits in your heart. Grief can be a forever kind of thing and while it will become easier to carry, the yearning to see, hug, and talk to your loved one again may never end.

————————————

If I'm honest, I sometimes struggle to write the words I know are tough to read. I wish I could share something more uplifting when it comes to loss and grief.

I wish I could make your deepest wishes come true and take your pain away.

But I can't. I can't fix your grief and I can't make promises that the journey of grief will be a skip through the daisy fields or that you will find gold at the end of the rainbow.

It breaks my heart because I know how hard the journey of grief is. I know what it feels like to miss someone so much it hurts.

People will ask me how long the pain of grief lasts. People desperately want to know if they will always feel this awful or if the feeling of missing their loved one will settle down and fade.

While I can't know how your journey will unfold, I can tell you the pain will dull but the missing never completely goes away.

You will always miss your loved one because love never ends. The love, grief, and sense of loss are a forever kind of thing.

It's impossible to forget or replace someone you love and regardless of how much time goes by, it's incredibly difficult to completely fill the deep void that now sits restlessly in your heart.

That's how grief works when loving another human being becomes part of your story. Love is eternal and so it makes sense that the grief you carry is eternal too.

One of the hardest things about loss is knowing you will never see, touch, hold, or talk to your loved one again in this lifetime. The thought of that hurts, and at times, it's a heartbreaking reality that's hard to accept.

People looking at your grief from the outside and through their own skewed lenses may have a difficult time understanding how painful this is for you. It's unfair of them to expect that you will hurry up and get over it. That's an impossible ask.

With that being said, you won't always feel as bad as you do right now. It won't always be as gut-wrenching nor will you feel as lost and hopeless as you do today. You will always miss your loved one, but over time, the missing will look different. Hopefully, it won't hurt as much and you will find more comfort in the love and less discomfort from the pain.

I'm not saying you won't have bad days when the missing is hard to shake off and the ache cuts deep. But hopefully it won't bring a tsunami of suffering like it once did or last as long.

And every time you miss your loved one, send them love and light.

A life-altering loss comes with so much change. As if losing a loved one isn't painful enough, the avalanche of secondary losses will knock you down and cover your heart with extra layers of pain and grief.

Grief *is* exhausting. And when you think about how hard loss and grief really are, feeling worn out makes perfect sense.

A significant loss changes your life and forces you to adjust to a life that looks nothing like it did before. Loss will tear apart and dismantle life piece by piece, and it's not just about grieving for your loved one. You will quickly realize you are grieving for so many other things.

Loss shakes everything loose and brings an avalanche of secondary losses that will quickly pile up; the weight of it all can take you down. Yet, secondary losses are not always recognized or acknowledged even though they create mountains of stress and extra layers of grief.

It's hard enough to navigate the grief you're carrying for your loved one, but to add the extra load of so many additional losses is overwhelming, and it can feel as if the grief is sucking the air right out of you.

The cumulative grief adds up and takes a heavy toll, and far too many grievers don't realize just how damaging secondary losses can be.

Secondary losses to be aware of might include:

Loss of relationships.

Loss of identity.

Loss of security and stability.

Loss of financial support.

Loss of the roles you played at home, work, and in the community.

Loss of help.

Loss of hope.

Loss of companionship.

Loss of your future plans and dreams.

Loss of your health.

I've barely scratched the surface of all the different ways loss shows up, but it's critical to be aware of secondary losses and how quickly they can stack up.

The grief you're experiencing for any of these losses is valid and needs to be processed and expressed.

Grief is relentless and it makes sense when grievers feel overwhelmed and fatigued. It's a lot to manage and a big ask for anyone.

Be kind to yourself. Take extra good care of your mind, body, and heart. Give yourself permission to grieve all of the losses that are slowly squeezing your heart in a vice. You will learn to adapt and adjust to all of the changes. Eventually, you will fold each and every loss into what feels like a different life, but it's important to recognize them first. It might help to reflect on this and make a list of all of the secondary losses you are trying to manage and carry.

I know it's a lot to process, and remember, it's okay to lean on others and it's okay to ask for help.

The anticipation of losing a loved one after a life-changing terminal diagnosis can lead to feelings of fear, pain, and grief long before your loved one dies and you are forced to say a final goodbye.

——————————

The beginning of the end of a loved one's life is heartbreaking and it can lead to grief long before they draw their last breath.

Regardless of time, the period before death arrives can be filled with fear and despair. It's a time of complex emotions and it can be difficult to know how to feel or what to expect.

People don't always recognize the grief that shows up long before the time of death. But anticipatory grief is real and it's important to acknowledge it and give yourself permission to grieve regardless of how much time is left.

Some people will survive for months or even years after a heartbreaking diagnosis. Others will last for no more than a few days or weeks. Time is irrelevant when it comes to grieving and it will be a time in your life that asks you to carry anxiety, fear, and pain.

If you're a caretaker for someone you care about and love, you will meet grief quickly, and it will be exhausting. You'll be forced to face the fact that your loved one is changing, slipping away, and that their life will come to an end. Anticipating a guaranteed loss is difficult.

As you grieve the inevitable, life continues to go on. The world keeps moving as if nothing is wrong. But something is wrong. You're slowly losing someone you love and there's nothing you can do to change it.

It's a painful burden to carry and it's often one that's carried in silence.

It's a time that can be overrun with extreme fatigue and guilt. Sometimes you pray for the suffering to end yet you are terrified of losing them. It's a confusing time that doesn't always come with much-needed understanding and support.

If you're dealing with a diagnosis, whether it's for yourself or a loved one, please honor the grief you're feeling. Take extra good care of yourself and give yourself permission to feel all your emotions and grieve.

Sit inside your pain and the grief you're carrying in your heart. Recognize the anger, hopelessness, exhaustion, sadness, and fear as valid emotions that need to move through you and with you from one day to the next.

Self-care is essential. It's okay to set boundaries and it's okay to ask for help.

I'm sorry if you're struggling under the weight of anticipatory grief. Please know your grief is valid and deserves to be seen and heard.

I'm sending you love and compassion as you walk this difficult journey.

Grief is exhausting and there will be days when it feels like a full-time job. A job that feels overwhelming and incredibly hard, because it is. Go easy on yourself and remember, if the only thing you are able to accomplish today is surviving, that's enough.

———————————

"I'm so exhausted all the time. I'm so tired it feels like I'm walking through cement and everything feels so heavy I just want to crawl into bed and sleep. Everything feels overwhelming and hard."

Do these words sound familiar to you? Have you felt so worn out it's difficult to function and keep up with the demands of life?

If so, you're not alone. Grievers often feel a deep fatigue that's hard to shake. And while society doesn't always get it, grief is exhausting and there will be days when it does feel like a never-ending, thankless job. A job that offers no formal training. A job that doesn't always provide much-needed support or breaks.

There are no deadlines to meet or standard operating procedures to follow, and all that's required of you changes from one day to the next.

There are no textbooks to study or manuals that teach you how to grieve. Yet, society expects everyone to figure it out as quickly as possible, get the job done, and move on.

But that's not how grief works. Grief is a full-time job and it's not a job you master in a few days or complete before you move on to something else.

Grief becomes part of daily life and while there will be days when the workload isn't as heavy, there will be days that feel so draining, it's challenging to manage everything.

Grievers typically don't grieve as a team or collaborate with others to complete the job. No one can grieve for you and you're the only expert in your personal grief journey. People can certainly support you and listen, but most of the hard work of grief must be done alone.

With that being said, it's important to find people you can lean on when the weight of grief feels too heavy. It's important to draw support from people who get it and will keep showing up without unrealistic expectations or demands you can't meet.

There's no such thing as doing the job of grieving wrong. There's no such thing as failing at grief or falling behind.

Self-care is critical and grievers need to take frequent breaks. If possible, take the day off once in a while.

Have mercy on yourself. If the only thing you do today is survive, that's okay. And whether you feel like it or not, you deserve credit for showing up every day and doing your best.

I know you don't always feel like you're doing a good job but you are and for every day you keep moving, you deserve to be recognized for trying. You deserve to know how much your efforts matter.

Survival, Self-Care, and Finding Your Way Forward

There is life after loss. You just have to be willing to open your heart to the possibilities and, with courage, choose to show up and embrace life again.

When someone you love dies, the pain of grief can feel overwhelming. And when grief takes over your life, it's easy to feel powerless and completely lost.

There will be days when everything feels too hard and the weight of grief is so heavy it's difficult to believe you will find a path forward, let alone find the good side of life again.

It's scary to loosen your grip and let go of the "before" as you step blindly into the unknown of a life that has changed so much. Most people don't have a clue about what to do when loss invades their lives. It can feel like you're wearing a blindfold as you struggle to navigate the complicated journey of grief.

There is so much being asked of you. So many unanswered questions. Everything seems coated with a thick layer of fear and uncertainty.

How could life not feel dark and hopeless for a while?

But here's the thing: It is possible to move forward and find purpose again even after someone you love dies.

So how do you move forward after loss?

I don't have all of the answers and your path forward may look very different than mine. There's no one way to do this thing called grief, but moving forward often begins with a desire to live a full life again—and lots of grace.

Grievers need an abundance of patience, curiosity, self-love, and self-compassion, especially when the rest of the world fails to understand and show up.

Moving forward requires a shift in perspective and a change in the way you talk to yourself. It takes changing your thinking from "What's the point?" or "I can't do this" to learning to integrate your loss and grief into your life.

There is life after loss but it's important to remember that your thoughts can hold great power over you. If you allow them to control you, they will take you prisoner and keep you trapped in the pain.

The smallest shifts in your thinking can open up a corridor to restore hope.

Awareness is key. Pay attention to how you talk to yourself and make an effort to discard words that hold you back or keep you stuck in a place you no longer want to be.

Stop saying the word *never.*

"I will never survive this."

"I will never find happiness again."

"This is my reality now and my life will never be good again."

Even if that's what you believe to be true right now, it's time for that word to leave your vocabulary.

Learning to live with a devastating loss means giving yourself permission to grieve, and it means cracking the door open just wide enough to step back into the world as you search for renewed purpose and meaning.

The journey of grief is, in part, about opening your heart, mind, and soul to all of the possibilities that lie on the other side of the darkness and being curious about how life could be in the months ahead.

Life after loss is within your reach but there will be days when it comes down to choice. You have to want to find healing and to grow around your grief. You have to want to push off the bottom of the deep end of the pool and swim back to the surface so you can breathe.

It's a slow process and it's not a race to win. But you have to be willing to show up, step onto the starting block, and *move*—even if it's one small step at a time.

Living a full life after loss is possible if you are willing to be honest with yourself and sit with your grief. It's important to feel all of your emotions instead of trying to outrun the pain.

Perhaps you're not there yet and everything feels impossible right now. Perhaps you don't want to believe it's real, and it feels safer to deny and pretend. Or perhaps you can't imagine fitting back into the world ever again.

I get it.

I'm not saying the journey forward is easy. There are no quick detours nor is there a magical antidote to the pain of grief, but trust me when I tell you that with time, the bitter taste of grief will fade. Eventually, you will start to recognize parts of the old you as you adapt to this new version of you and your life.

Your energy will slowly return and as you dig your way out of the rubble, you will discover new pathways that can propel you forward.

Try filling your day with healthy distractions and spending time doing things you are passionate about. Find a new hobby, help others, and volunteer. Spend time in nature, take a class, immerse yourself in a project, or surround yourself with kind and supportive friends.

As counterintuitive as it might feel, it's easier to live a full life after loss if you're willing to embrace and own your grief. It's important to take the armor off and surrender to it. Stop hiding how you really feel and get rid of the clutter that's clogging up your heart, mind, and home.

I know it can be difficult to believe any of this in the early days after a life-changing loss. It can be a challenge to find the desire to search for hope under the debris. As the mountain of grief looms in front of you, it's hard to know where to start or how to begin. Sometimes the first step is the hardest one but it's necessary to take that first step toward new beginnings and the possibility of healing.

You can do this. Make the choice and, step by step, you can move closer to a life offering you a sense of purpose and joy. Stay the course, be curious, and remember that anything is possible.

There will be times when you feel like you've tried everything to lessen the pain. Yoga. Meditation. Prayer. Journaling. Going outside for a walk. Talking to a counselor or with a friend. Support groups. Crying until there are no tears left to cry. Screaming at the world. Distracting yourself with work or trying to sleep away the pain. No matter how hard you try, you still find yourself struggling. Please remember, it's not because you're doing anything wrong and it's not because you're weak. It's because grief is sometimes relentless after the permanence of loss sets in. So if you have days when nothing seems to provide relief, trust the process and don't give up. Tomorrow you can try again.

———————————

There will be days when no amount of work or effort dulls the pain of grief and you wake up feeling as awful as you did the day before.

I know how frustrating that feels.

But as discouraging as it is, there are no quick fixes when it comes to loss and grief. You can't speed up the process. There's only time, patience, and loving yourself through the pain.

You can't rush through grief even though society expects you to. Regardless of how much time has gone by, if the loss is big enough, grief will stubbornly dig in its heels and remind you it's here to stay.

There will be moments that test your ability to heal, and sometimes you will feel too exhausted to do the hard work grief requires you to do.

Grief will stretch your soul in gut-wrenching ways and, as deflating as it can be, there will be times when nothing helps and the pain of loss will break your heart all over again.

Please don't be discouraged. You're not doomed to a lifetime of unmanageable suffering. While there's no one antidote for a broken heart and you may always carry grief with you, there are things you can do to help ease the pain.

Movement and exercise are good for the mind, body, and soul. Breathing in fresh air or getting outside for a daily dose of sunshine can help too.

Write or scribble your feelings in a journal. Talk to a counselor, family member, or friend. Take your dog for a walk. Listen to relaxing music, surrender, and take a nap. Watch your favorite show, garden, organize a closet, or listen to a favorite podcast.

Volunteer. Paint. Sing in the shower. Dance. Go to a movie, take a class, plan a weekend getaway with friends, cook your favorite meal, or write a letter to your loved one and say all that was left unsaid.

Any of these can provide the gift of distraction and bring moments of relief. They will help you to weather the daily grind of grieving a loss that left your life in shambles.

You will have days when you're stuck on an emotional roller coaster. Days when it's a challenge to stand upright and despite your best effort, it's difficult to function at all.

You may have days when it feels like nothing helps.

Be extra kind to yourself on those extra hard days. It doesn't mean you're failing at grieving, nor does it mean you will feel like this forever or that you are weak.

There's no pass-fail here. You're a brave human who knows the pain of great loss and as frustrating as it is, there will be those days when nothing seems to help and the only thing you can do is get through the day and survive.

Hold on, and if you're having a day when nothing seems to work, take a step back and give yourself permission to just sit inside your grief and pain. As counterintuitive as that might feel, sometimes it's the only thing that helps.

You will survive this, even though it's hard to believe right now. The sharp edges of grief will dull and with time they will not cut so deeply.

Remember, if something didn't help today, you can get up tomorrow and try again.

Sometimes you just need to sit inside the grief and pain. Absorb it and feel it. It's not going anywhere and there will be moments when it's the only thing that makes sense after you lose someone you love.

———————————

The pain of grief is often one of the most brutal and difficult things human beings are forced to carry and endure.

It's a monumental struggle and there are no quick or easy escape routes when grief traps you in the pain of your loss.

As much as people try to ignore its presence, the urgent and sometimes all-consuming pain of grief runs with wild abandon and there will be moments when everything feels out of control.

You can try to pretend it's not there, but grief won't lay dormant for long, and eventually, it will demand to be acknowledged and heard.

I know it can feel counterintuitive to sit inside the pain. Who the hell wants to hang out with grief and feel so sad all the time? I didn't want to and it took me a long time to face my grief let alone welcome it and sit with it.

But this is what grief will ask all of us to do.

As difficult as it is, grief asks us to sit and just be with all the hard feelings that plant deep roots inside our hearts. Grief will ask you to dip your foot in the water, one toe at a time. And slowly, you will submerge your body, heart, and soul as you learn how to absorb the grief that now lives inside you.

Sometimes there are no words for the emotional pain and it can feel easier to manage a headache or broken bone. But there's comfort to be found inside of the pain because it's a way to stay connected to your loved one and the life you lived before.

Your grief isn't going anywhere. It's part of you now and as much as it hurts to sit inside it, it's important to embrace it and carry it with you.

I worked closely with a woman who lost her dad before her wedding. She was crushed and for a very long time she couldn't face the pain. Megan tried to ignore her grief and distract herself with work. She pretended she was fine even though she was falling apart inside.

That worked for a while, but eventually, grief caught up with her. Her feelings became too big and the grief bubbled up and burst, causing her more grief and pain. Her relationships and work suffered, and her health broke down.

By the time Megan reached out for help, her world had shrunk so much, she didn't know who she was or how to function anymore.

Megan needed to reset and reclaim her right to grieve. She needed to learn how to sit with the grief and own all of her feelings regardless of how painful they were. Once Megan was able to peel back the layers and face the pain, she slowly started to heal and rebuild.

It's true that grief isn't something to be fixed or cured. It doesn't work to run from it or pretend it doesn't exist. You can't outrun something if it becomes a permanent fixture in your life and heart.

As much as it hurts, it's sometimes necessary to retreat within and just sit with the pain. To run toward all that feels so broken and let it break you even more. Sometimes everything has to fall apart before you can start to pick up the pieces and rebuild.

It may be hard to see a clear path forward right now but it's there, and while it might be hidden under a dense blanket of grief and pain, you will find a way to forge ahead. Remember, the pain doesn't have to control you forever and eventually, it will ease.

I can't tell you when that will be. It's your journey and you must find your own way one step at a time. But you will survive and when you least expect it, light will find its way back into your heart.

Life can feel so unfair. Sometimes things happen that are so awful it can feel like all of the emotions drain right out of you, leaving you empty and numb inside. Don't worry. Sometimes you have to empty everything out to fill your heart back up again.

It's really hard. All of it. Tend to the parts of you that feel broken, but have faith that not everything is broken in your life. There is still good to be found. You just have to be open to searching for it when your grief settles down and the pain subsides. And it will.

Grief doesn't make you different
from other people in the world.
Grief makes you human in the most
sacred of ways, and allowing yourself
to fall apart even though the rest
of the world expects you to hold
it together is an act of bravery.

One of the saddest things about loss and grief is when the grieving feel like they are suddenly different from everyone else and struggling to fit in.

Sitting at the table of grief can feel like one of the loneliest places on earth, especially when you feel like you've lost your place in the world along with parts of your identity.

Society will tell you that to be brave means sucking it up, being strong, staying positive in the face of adversity, and—with a smile on your face—getting over it.

But that's not true. You don't get over it. Getting over a painful death isn't like getting over failing your driver's test or missing your flight. Death isn't something to overcome. It's something you must learn to live with, and frankly, you will constantly be searching for ways to adapt to living without your loved one.

The true essence of what it means to be brave after loss has blown your life apart is, in part, finding the courage to face the pain regardless of what the rest of the world thinks.

Sometimes, bravery isn't bold and loud. It's the smallest of acts, and in the face of grief, it's incredibly brave to let your heart break. To be brave is to cry and fall apart when you miss your beloved so much it feels like you're going to explode.

Bravery is being vulnerable enough to fall down as often as you need but then finding a way to get back up and try again.

To be brave is to tell the truth and not live in fear of showing the world your grief and pain. It's finding the courage to ask for help when your energy is depleted and you can't do it alone anymore.

To be brave is to meet yourself where you are every single day instead of trying to please everyone else or trying to be someone you're not after grief has rearranged everything.

It doesn't matter how much time has drifted by. If you continue to have days when life is a struggle, it's okay. There's nothing wrong with saying no and choosing to put you and your grief first. You don't have to fake it all the time, and from where I stand, you are incredibly brave to keep going and keep giving yourself permission to be human and grieve.

Undoubtedly, grievers are some of the bravest, kindest, most compassionate people I know. We are all hurting and grief doesn't separate us or make us different from one another. Grief unites us and together we can survive the pain.

Everyone who grieves must find a way to survive in a brave new world. You've got this and I believe in you.

If you do one thing today, be kind to yourself. You're grieving and you deserve kindness, compassion, and love.

———————————————

Loss is so hard and there will be moments when grief is all-consuming and feels as if it might swallow you whole.

Our minds, bodies, and hearts take a beating after a life-changing loss, and while we grieve for a reason, there will be days when it takes a huge toll.

I know life is busy and, whether you're grieving or not, it doesn't skip a beat or slow down—even after loss shakes everything up.

Grief is exhausting and the demands of life don't seem to care but it's imperative that you find pockets of time to slow down and catch your breath.

It's important to carve out plenty of time for rest and self-care. Your well-being depends on it and if you do nothing else today, please be gentle with your grieving heart. Give yourself lots of compassion and be extra kind to *you*.

I can't think of anyone who deserves love and kindness more than someone who is grieving an overwhelming loss. But the world can be an unforgiving place when it comes to grief, and sometimes it's necessary to course correct and put yourself first.

When you're grieving, you don't always get the love and support you need. People can be judgmental and unkind at a time when you need kindness the most. You can't always control what others say and do, but you can choose how you treat yourself.

And if someone is being unkind, it's okay to walk away and protect your heart. If possible, surround yourself with people who bring love, understanding, and compassion into your heart and home. That's what you deserve when loss has brought so much pain into your world.

Even when others struggle to be kind, you can be kind to yourself. Sometimes you need to have your own back and put yourself first. And when you find yourself sitting alone with your grief, surrender to it and have faith that, while different, life won't always feel this insufferable.

Please be kind to yourself.

Give yourself permission to say no.
Cancel plans. Stay in bed. Cry. Laugh.
Wear pajamas all day. Be angry. Feel
overwhelmed. Be sad. Feel sorry for
yourself. Skip the party. Sit alone in
silence. Go to the party. Ask for help.
Let your heart break. Allow exhaustion
to sink into your bones and take a
nap. Dance. Curl up in a cozy blanket
and do nothing at all. Expect more
from others. Surrender to the pain.
Give yourself permission to grieve.

What do you need today? It's a simple question, but when grief becomes part of your daily life, it can be a difficult one to answer. Grievers don't always know what they want or need and, just like grief, your needs and wants will continue to shift and change.

Grief is erratic and it's in a constant state of ebb and flow. Emotions come and emotions go. Thankfully, no feeling lasts forever even though it can feel like some of the most painful feelings will never go away.

It's impossible to screw up grief because there's no wrong way to grieve. I will keep reminding you that the only way to grieve is your way. It's a sacred journey and everyone will grieve differently.

Keeping that in mind, most grievers feel stuck at some point and it doesn't help when society expects the grieving to act and behave in certain ways. To return to the hectic demands of life long before they are ready.

People sometimes feel shunned as they struggle to fit back into a world that doesn't understand their grief. And regretfully, grievers often conceal their pain while trying to grieve in ways that are acceptable to people sitting on the sidelines of their journey, having never walked in a griever's shoes.

But grief doesn't operate that way. There's no perfect way to grieve, and honestly, grievers need to push back and take control of their own journey despite what the outside world believes.

It's time for you to give yourself permission to feel all that you need to feel even though your emotions might run wildly out of control.

Give yourself permission to do something out of the ordinary. Something that allows you to escape, even just for a moment, from the limitations others have put on you and your grieving heart.

The journey of grief can be grueling at best, and it's more than okay to put yourself first and honor your needs.

Say no. Connect with others who get it. Sit in the silence and comfort of your bedroom. Cry, and if it means sobbing out loud, go for it. Laugh until your stomach hurts.

Take a hot, relaxing shower or bubble bath. Or skip the shower if you don't feel like taking one today and let your hair be a mess. Feel sorry for yourself. Let the sadness in. Do something that brings you joy. If possible, stay in your pajamas all day. Get up and go for a long walk in nature. Go back to bed. Choose to be defiant and not a victim.

Cancel plans. Make plans. Go to the party. Leave the party early. Feel overwhelmed and do nothing at all. Order takeout for breakfast, lunch, and dinner if you don't feel like cooking. Be angry. Let the laundry pile up. Write in your journal. Dance. Paint. Have a movie marathon. Volunteer. Do something that brings you purpose and meaning. Call a friend. Sip on a cup of coffee or tea and enjoy a donut or two.

Take the day off and just grieve.

Whatever it is, give yourself permission to do it without feeling any regret or guilt.

I know life demands a lot and it's challenging to do some of the things you really want to do. But grief asks so much of you and it's important to try and find time to do something that fills your empty cup again.

Climbing the mountain of grief that's set up camp at the base of your life might feel like an impossible task. The voice inside your head might be saying you will never reach the top.

But I want you to remember that anything is possible. There's always going to be another mountain to climb and grief is an uphill battle for a long time. But if you keep inching up that mountain, even if you have to crawl, you will get there.

You don't have to do it all today, but when you're ready, the tiniest of action steps can help you to reach for the stars and climb out of the pain.

Give yourself permission—and if it's a stay-in-your-pajamas-and-eat-an-entire-bag-of-donuts kind of day, you have my vote to do so without guilt.

Grief is personal and it's important to grieve in whatever way feels right for you. Meet yourself right where you are every single day and stop allowing the people in your life to dictate or demand that you meet them where they need and want you to be. Your well-being depends on it.

———————————

Meet yourself right where you are. I can't say this enough because it's so important when it comes to loss and grief.

We exist in a world that's constantly trying to candy-coat the tough stuff that happens in life. To downplay just how bad it really is. To minimize the pain of a loss that shredded your world into a million pieces and then left you to grieve alone as if it's not that big of a deal.

But your grief is a big deal. Don't let anyone tell you it's not.

Sadly, there will always be people who don't understand your grief. To be frank, there are people who don't want to. It's too uncomfortable; your loss can rattle people and remind them that life doesn't come with guarantees.

There are millions of people grieving in the world yet society tries to lock grief in a box and throw away the key. It feels safer to hide it away and pretend it doesn't matter or exist.

But grief does matter and it does exist. Painful, terrible things happen, sometimes in the most tragic and traumatic of ways. Grief can't be confined and no lock is strong enough to keep grief from breaking free.

Grief should never be ignored and it's unfair for the outside world to expect anyone who knows the pain of loss to shake off the pain and get over it.

People don't get it and some will try to discourage you from grieving and place unrealistic demands on you. There will be people who can't meet you where you are, and, while it's unfair, they'll ask you to meet them where they are and want you to be.

Don't fold and give in to the ignorance of others. The only thing that matters right now is you and your grief. You don't have to keep trying so hard to protect and please everyone else.

The essence of good self-care after loss is learning to believe in yourself again. Be confident, speak your truth, and don't worry about what the rest of the world thinks about you and your grief.

Society will try to derail you and pull you back into a world that no longer fits the same for you. But you're the captain of this journey and no one gets to navigate but you.

Listen to your own heart and stop listening to the outside noise. Be gentle with yourself and be patient as you try to find your bearings again.

Your grief *is* a big deal and one of the best things you can do is ignore the unrealistic expectations of others and focus on your needs as you carry your grief forward.

Meet yourself right where you are every single day and resist the urge to suppress your feelings and hide them away. Honoring your grief is where the possibility of finding hope, joy, and meaning again resides.

This is your life and you get to live, love, and grieve on your own terms.

Self-care is one of the first things to go after loss tears everything down. The early days of grief can be so disorienting, it's easy to forget to take care of yourself and do the most basic of things. But self-care is vital to your well-being and to weathering the storms of loss. If you do one thing today, take care of yourself.

As difficult as it may be, it's so important for you to figure out how to take care of yourself after loss.

While it may feel unreasonable or contradictory to take care of yourself, it's imperative for your well-being while carrying the heavy weight of grief.

Some people feel guilty and selfish but taking care of yourself is part of living a healthy and full life, even after loss.

Putting guilt aside for a moment, self-care is an essential part of the healing process when it comes to physical health and emotional wounds.

It's hard if not impossible to operate if you're exhausted and unwell.

Taking care of yourself may be the farthest thing from your mind right now and trust me when I say I understand. It's normal to wrap yourself in a cocoon of sorts and struggle to do much of anything, let alone practice good self-care.

But it's necessary, and honestly, there's no compromise when it comes to grief and taking care of yourself. And sometimes that means putting yourself first. You can't effectively take care of others if you don't first take care of yourself. And who, may I ask, is taking care of *you*?

Years ago, I worked as a flight attendant for Northwest Airlines. One of the first things they taught us was the importance of putting on your own oxygen mask first. You can't provide assistance to a loved one sitting next to you unless you're able to breathe.

I've learned that this metaphor applies to so many things in life, especially when it comes to grief and self-care.

You're a work in progress and you don't have to figure everything out today. But today is the perfect time to step up and take better care of yourself moving forward. It's never too late to start, and your well-being is counting on it.

I know how overwhelming that can feel, but you don't have to cook a gourmet meal or run a marathon. It's not about getting a massage, facial, or manicure. Good self-care is sometimes about saying no to others and saying yes to yourself.

It's not always about taking care of others: It's about taking care of yourself. It's about choosing you in your greatest time of need. It's not selfish to put yourself first if you can. You are worthy of the care your heart, mind, and body require after loss.

Be reasonable and start with a small and realistic goal.

Do the best you can, even if your best is getting out of bed and standing in the shower for five minutes. It's a start (and there's nothing like a hot shower when you feel exhausted and sad). Perhaps it's returning one phone call or responding to a few texts. Or maybe it's giving yourself permission to cry or talking to a trusted friend. Perhaps it's as simple as taking a five-minute walk or finding the energy to weed your garden and soak up some sun. Self-care is about getting plenty of rest, nourishing and moving your body, drinking plenty of water, and avoiding things that do more harm than good.

Whatever it is, give yourself grace and know that for today it's enough. The more you honor your well-being and take care of yourself in the most basic of ways, the quicker you will find energy and strength to move forward in life and manage your grief. Your mind, body, and heart will guide you and tell you what they need. Your job is to listen and do what's being asked of you, even when it feels hard.

Please take care and put your oxygen mask on first. Your healing and well-being depend on it.

Healing after loss doesn't mean your grief completely disappears nor does it mean you won't feel sad or carry a deep ache in your heart. And the truth is, there may be parts of you that never completely heal because missing your loved one will never go away.

Healing is a word that means different things to different people. Some people believe you can heal from loss with time, patience, and love. For others, healing feels impossible and it's hard to believe they will ever heal after a loved one dies.

Everyone grieves differently and you have the right to your feelings, thoughts, and beliefs. You get to determine how your personal grief journey will evolve and unfold.

Grief settles into your heart and bones. It can feel like life will never feel okay again, and it's understandable to question if all that feels so broken will heal.

Healing from a heartbreaking loss isn't the same as healing or recovering from a bad cold. It's not as simple as getting extra rest, drinking plenty of orange juice, taking medicine, and eating a bowl of hot chicken noodle soup.

Sometimes healing after loss requires you to face the pain and break open a little bit more. Sometimes it's the breaking that helps you to climb out of the abyss and piece yourself back together again even though you will be a different version of who you once were.

Grief becomes a companion of sorts after a loved one dies. It resides in the heart and while the flames of grief will wane, they may never completely burn out.

Keeping that in mind, the question of how to heal when grief lasts forever is a fair and honorable one.

There's no right or wrong answer. Everything you experience will be personal to you.

Perhaps there's a middle ground. Perhaps it's about redefining what healing means to you and learning to accept the possibility that some parts of your grieving heart may not completely heal. But with resilience and the inherent will to survive, you will discover you can heal just enough to move forward and find joy in your life again. And the truth is, it starts with wanting to heal.

Healing doesn't mean you will ever forget nor will you leave your grief behind. It doesn't mean you won't ever feel lonely, angry, or sad. Healing doesn't mean you will completely fill the void that now rests in your heart nor does it mean you won't always yearn to see your loved one again.

Part of what it means to heal is to learn to integrate grief into your new and different life. It means finding a way to manage the pain of grief so it doesn't leave you feeling exhausted and gutted all the time. It means focusing on the love more than the pain and having moments of peace.

Healing means finding deeper ways to connect to your loved one even though death has created a divide. It means rediscovering meaning and purpose in your life and focusing on what matters most.

And while you might be forever changed by the experience of loss, healing means learning to love and accept the person you've become.

Laughter and joy may not come as easily as before, but healing parts of yourself will create more space for love and light so things don't always feel so hopeless and dark.

I recognize that healing won't look the same for everyone and no one has the right to tell you what it means for you. But it's my hope that healing will find its way to you and that your ability to experience beauty, peace, and joy will be restored.

Those who have walked through the fires of loss and carry the flames of grief in their heart know how important it is to show up for others with compassion, grace, and love.

———————————

Sadly, the grieving often feel isolated and alone. They feel abandoned by the people they thought would be there through thick and thin. People they thought they could count on when awful stuff happens in life.

Sometimes validation and compassion show up and sometimes they don't. And when support is nowhere to be found, it's disappointing and it hurts.

With that being said, I've found that grievers are some of the most loving, kind, and compassionate people I know. Through their own journey of loss and grief, they instinctively know what others so badly need.

Once you walk through the fires of loss and carry the flames of grief, you change. As hard as you might try, there's no turning back.

Perspectives change. Things that once mattered no longer hold your attention. The days of empty and hollow chitchat are gone. And it's hard to fill the painful hole that now rests in your soul.

The grieving become more aware of the fragility of life and it becomes easier to see the pain that others carry. Grievers have been there, which is why they can see past the bullshit.

Grief creates a universal bond through our shared experiences of loss, and suddenly, you can understand another's sorrow and pain as if it's your very own.

Perhaps you didn't get the support and compassion you so desperately needed and yet you feel pulled to help others in their time of need. You know how lonely and isolating grief can be, and if you're anything like me, you don't want anyone else to feel stranded in despair, left to grieve completely alone.

So for anyone reading this who gets it, thank you for your kind heart. Thank you for your compassion and offering your shoulder for others to lean on. Your grace, compassion, and brave heart are gifts in a world that's full of hurting souls.

I wish you didn't know these truths and I wish you didn't personally know the pain of loss and grief.

We are traveling this road together even though we are apart, and giving compassion and grace to others will make a huge difference to anyone feeling abandoned after loss.

Kindness goes a long way and will make a difference in the world but please remember to give yourself compassion and be kind to your own broken heart. And hopefully, someone will show you kindness too.

You matter. Your grief matters. And from one griever to another, I know you've walked through fire to get here and I'm proud of you.

The truth is, it takes a village to get through the tough stuff in life. It doesn't have to be a big village but we all need people to help hold us up when life, loss, and grief knock us down.

I'm sure you've heard the phrase, "It takes a village."

The phrase originated in Africa and it conveys the message that it takes many people to raise a child. To provide a safe, healthy environment for children to feel secure and to flourish in life.

To say "It takes a village" when it comes to surviving what feels like an unsurvivable loss couldn't be more relevant and true.

While it's true that the hardest work of grief must be done alone and no one can carry your grief for you, grief creates an unbreakable bond with others who have traveled the road of grief before you, with you, and after you.

Grief is lonely and it's a solo journey that's personal to you, but that doesn't mean you have to shut yourself away from the rest of the world or shrink your world down so small that no one can help you.

We all need to belong and human beings need companionship and connection to survive. People are wired for attachment and after loss takes so much away, the grieving long for and need a community that stands together and shares their sorrow and pain.

It does take a village to help grievers feel safe and secure. To have people to count on, lean on, and reach out to when the pain is too heavy to bear.

Grievers need to connect with people who can cut through all the nonsense and crap. To dust off the cobwebs and recognize the grief and pain because they too have walked on the edges of hell— even though no two losses are the same and everyone's hell will look different.

It doesn't have to be a big village. Sometimes your village may house one or two kind souls you've come to know and trust. Other villages may be much larger and cast a wider net. Regardless of how many people reside in your village, it's important to find people to connect with and people who are willing to step into each other's pain.

No one can take your grief away. But finding kinship and connecting with others who get it can ease the burden, provide a much-needed cushion to absorb some of the pain, and help you to feel less alone.

Grief moves in us and through us, and if you connect with other grievers, it will move between you with love. You deserve to feel safe and supported when grief upends your life. You deserve to feel like you belong and to be surrounded with unconditional support and care.

Consider me and the pages of this book to be part of your village. A place where your grief is safe and you feel understood with love.

It may not feel like it right now, but you will get through this and you will survive. You will. And part of surviving is finding the courage to keep going even when you feel destroyed inside. It's about wanting to feel better and choosing to do the hard work it takes to rise above a loss that's changed your life and who you are. You will get through this and survive. You will.

———————————

A devastating loss takes the roots you've carefully planted over the years and rips them right out of the ground you once stood on. The ground that suddenly crumbles beneath you is like a giant sinkhole, and the foundation you believed would always be there gives way under the weight of a loss that destroyed parts of the life you built and loved. A loss that changed your world in immeasurable ways.

How do you survive that? How do you climb out of the hole that pulled you and so many things you care about down into the dark space of the unknown?

The soul-shattering experience of loss changes people. You are no longer the same person you were at the beginning of your story—but it's important to remember that even now, that story's ending has yet to be written.

A life-altering loss can lead to emotional bankruptcy and it's difficult to find your footing in the aftermath of loss. And frankly speaking, the hard work of grief will ask you to do things you never wanted to do or thought you could.

It's unforgiving and exhausting work, and while the loss itself is painfully hard, choosing to fight and claw your way back to living is one of the hardest things to do after loss rearranges everything.

But if you don't make the choice to push off the bottom of that deep, dark hole and climb out, you will stay trapped in between the life you miss and the new life that awaits you.

To move forward after loss, you must be willing to let go and shed parts of yourself. Parts you never imagined giving up or living without.

Stepping into a new way of being is scary and it's human to look in the rearview mirror of your life and want to turn back. But turning back won't help you. You can't go back to a place that no longer exists. At least not in the same way as before.

There's only moving forward, and inch by inch you will return to a new version of yourself and arrive to a place that looks different but can be beautiful again.

It's challenging work, and relearning to live after loss isn't about taking one big leap forward but rather it's a series of the tiniest movements fueled by choice. It's about doing things you don't want to do, and even if it means crawling, you do it because it's the only way to move beyond the intense pain and survive.

There will be days when you can't. When you're too exhausted to move and it takes too much energy to get up. To drag yourself out of bed takes a herculean effort, and in those moments, you get to say, "Not today," if you can.

It's okay to have days when you just can't do what life requires of you, but please don't give up. Stay the course and see it through. Trust yourself and trust the process. When you're ready, you will pull yourself out and find the courage to keep going.

You have to keep choosing to move forward and sometimes it's choosing inside of one moment at a time. It means choosing to never settle and choosing to face the unknown and not be paralyzed by fear. It means choosing to not let loss and grief destroy you or the chance to find happiness again.

Sometimes it's necessary to choose to do hard things even though you're exhausted and broken inside. And when you free-fall backward, you need to find the courage to mend your heart and get back up again.

You will learn a lot about yourself in the days, weeks, and months after loss crushes you. You will inevitably learn to dig deep and find the strength you need to survive and keep moving.

I had a client who was feeling trapped in her grief and pain. She was stuck in a deep canyon that divided her life before and after the loss of her husband. She felt trapped and desperate to find her way out.

She *wanted* to feel better and she *wanted* to find joy again. Honestly, that's half the battle and if you're willing to let grief crack you open and do the hard work, you will find your way forward regardless of how long it takes. And when she made the choice to do just that, she discovered a new path toward healing.

My client is still grieving and sad. She will never stop missing her husband and some days she takes a step forward and then five steps back. But she keeps trying and even if it's the smallest of things, she chooses to do something meaningful and productive every day. She has learned that she can do hard things, and she learned it starts with exceptional self-care.

And so can you. Little things add up over time. Start small and set the tiniest of goals. Perhaps it's as simple as spending five minutes responding to emails, cleaning out a drawer, or taking a ten-minute walk. Eventually, the small things will grow and expand. Eventually, you will move further than you dreamed was possible.

Loss and grief are going to suck no matter what you choose to do and it's so important to keep trying even when it feels too hard.

It's not always what happens to us but how we choose to react and respond to what happens. Even when your life has completely changed and you're feeling beat up, it comes down to making the decision to move forward and live again.

I'm not minimizing how hard any of this is and I understand how easy it is to fall into the pit of doom feeling like you can't possibly do life without your loved one.

I understand that you may feel like you won't get through this or survive. That you're destined to live a life of sorrow and pain.

But you will get through this and survive. You will.

Survival is about choosing and wanting to feel better, tapping into bravery and building on the resilience human beings carry deep inside their hearts.

Bravery isn't about winning a huge fight on the battlefield of loss. Bravery shines in the smallest of ways, and sometimes, it's about surrendering to your grief.

You can't control what others do but you can control what you do from one day to the next. And that includes taking care of yourself.

You won't function the same way you did before and things you used to do with ease may feel extra hard at first.

Resilience isn't about snapping back into the same life or the same shape you were before. Dr. Lucy Hone, author of *Resilient Grieving: Finding Strength and Embracing Life after a Loss That Changes Everything*, defines resilience as "the capacity to cope with, endure, withstand, steer through, and over time recover from disruption, challenge, loss, and change."

We are changed by the many experiences encountered in life and nothing changes us more than a devastating loss. A new version of yourself will slowly emerge and it's about finding ways to live comfortably in your different life while holding grief carefully in your heart.

It takes grit and grace to rebuild and I know it feels like everything is broken. But part of surviving is learning to open your eyes and discover those things that aren't broken.

You're still capable of caring about others, loving family and friends, giving back to society, improving your physical health, and finding things that give your life purpose and meaning again.

Choose to change what you can and let go of the things you can't. Dr. Hone writes, "Resilient people are good at choosing where they put their attention. They typically manage to focus on the things that they can change, and somehow accept the things that they can't."

I know grief has hijacked your life and I know how hopeless everything can feel. But human beings are built to survive and you will too. You can do hard things.

One of the first things people lose after a heartbreaking loss upends their life is hope. It can feel like all hope is gone forever and it will never be found again. But that's not true. Death is permanent but the loss of hope is temporary. It's patiently waiting in the corners of your broken heart until you're ready to reach for it again. There's always something to hope for even if it's hoping to survive or find a little joy.

A devastating loss interrupts life in ways no one can predict or see coming. Suddenly, life looks different and one of the many things that quickly disappear is hope.

The grieving mind struggles to find hope and it's normal to believe hope will never be found again.

It's easy to feel hopeless as you wander around feeling lost and in shock. Everything looks bleak and gray after loss drains the color out of your soul and life.

No one tells you how much loss and grief hurt. But it does hurt in the most gut-wrenching ways.

There will be days when it feels like the pain has emptied every last bit of hope out of your heart. Days when you feel so empty and numb, it's hard to feel much of anything at all.

The life you have come to know and love looks like a wasteland as you search through the debris and anything familiar is nowhere to be found.

I know it feels hopeless in the early days, weeks, and months after loss but I want you to know that, while hope is fleeting, you will find hope again.

We all need hope to get through the darkest of storms and survive. Hope is like oxygen and it's hope that can slowly breathe life back into our wounded hearts.

As hard as it is, death is permanent. But loss of hope is temporary, and hope is never far away. When you feel lost and like you won't get through the pain, searching for hope is a good place to start.

Hope is the bridge connecting what was to what is. It's a light that shines in the darkness and propels you forward, holding your hand every step of the way.

Hope will pull you back from the edge of the cliff before you fall.

Loss is painful and the path forward can feel like a daunting journey to take. But please remember there's always something to hope for even if it's hoping to find purpose or survive another day.

Don't give up, and start with one small hope at a time. Perhaps a good place to start is being hopeful it's possible to live a full life again.

Returning to life after a devastating loss is really hard. But life has a way of pulling you along with it whether you are ready or not. You will find your footing again in what will feel like a new and different world, and as impossible as it might feel, you will slowly return and rebuild.

———————————

A catastrophic loss of any kind is devastating and it can feel like everything you know and love has been destroyed in its path.

There will be days when it feels impossible to come back from the wreckage and move forward in life.

I get it. When loss strikes, it's easy to feel defeated and it's challenging to stand back up when grief knocks you down.

Life has asked way too much of you and I wish you didn't have to know this deep and searing pain. I wish grief hadn't pulled up alongside you and I wish I could somehow take your pain away.

Undoubtedly, coming back from a loss that's changed your life and who you are is incredibly hard. It will gut you and there will be moments when it feels like loss has stolen everything from you and there's nothing left.

I understand the moments that bring hopelessness and despair and it's easy to hit a wall and get stuck in your grief. But I want you to remember that there's always something left to hold on to—even if it's the powerful force of love.

Life will keep moving and it will pull you along. Regardless of how much time passes or how impossible everything feels.

It's possible to come back from the ruins and return to life. And as a fellow griever recently shared with me, "My heart is broken, but I'm still here. Here to remember and honor my loved one. Here to be part of this world. There's always something to hope for and honestly, life and love are everything."

For those of us left behind, it's possible to live life again. It's possible to rebuild. It won't be easy, especially when everything looks and feels different than before.

People will tell you to take it one day at a time but sometimes coming back feels so overwhelming, it's necessary to take it slower and breathe through one moment at a time.

I know it may be hard to believe but you can and will come back. And while nothing will look or feel exactly the same and you will always feel the absence of your loved one, it's possible to find joy and peace again when you're ready.

So when you're struggling to find hope or come back to living life, try to be curious. Search for the realm of possibilities that lie ahead for you even though it may mean experiencing life with grief in your heart.

You don't have to figure everything out today. Coming back takes time. Start small and be patient with yourself. Ask for help when it feels overwhelming and like it's just too much.

There are millions of grieving hearts in the world struggling to find their way back just like you. Find safety and connection in the grief community and know you're not completely alone.

Coming back from the unthinkable may feel impossible to you right now and my heart aches for you and with you. Loss will ask you to do impossible things and some days the grief you carry will feel relentless and take your breath away. But you're more resilient than you think and with time, you will find your way. Because truth be told, you deserve to live a full and happy life again—even though it will look different than before.

Don't ever apologize for struggling to come back. Sometimes the hardest part is returning to a life that no longer feels the same.

And as you return to life and fight to rebuild, know I'm cheering you on every step of the way.

In the early days of grief, when the pain is most fresh and intense, it's hard to imagine ever finding joy again. But when you're ready it is possible. The human heart can build resilience and has enough space to hold both grief and joy. It can take time to get there, but remember that grief doesn't have to be an either-or experience. It's never black-and-white. Grief and joy can walk through life side by side even when life feels heavy and dark. Find the "and," because you deserve a little bit of joy.

A painful loss can leave you feeling emptied from the inside out. It will stretch your soul in unimaginable ways and the grief you now carry will ask you to walk to the edge of ruin as you fight to keep from falling into the void. It comes with so many different emotions that collide into the life you're so desperately trying to live even though loss tore some of it down.

In the early days, weeks, and months following a devastating loss, there's no such thing as finding a cup that's half empty or half full. The cup is there but in the beginning, the cup of your heart often overflows with pain, sadness, anger, confusion, uncertainty, fear, anguish, shock, and guilt. It's a jumbled mess of emotions and it can feel impossible to swim through the debris and stay afloat.

So much about the grief experience is overwhelming and it's understandable if you feel like you will never feel okay again. The idea of finding happiness might feel like it's a million miles away.

Even if you do feel happy, it can conflict with what you think you *should* be feeling. Guilt often casts a shadow over good feelings like peace and joy.

Somehow people feel like it's wrong to feel happy and grieve at the same time. Human beings are conditioned to believe that grieving is an either-or experience and sometimes grievers instinctively close the door on happiness, believing it's wrong.

But grief is a multidimensional process and it's rarely black-and-white. It's possible to carry both positive and negative emotions, and you need to let go of the guilt and give yourself permission to feel both.

It's possible for light *and* beauty to peek through the cracks of everything that feels so ugly and dark. It's possible to both laugh *and* cry. To feel happy *and* sad. To find peace in the middle of the chaos. It's possible to hold space for both grief *and* joy.

If you're struggling to find the "and," I understand. But I want you to remember it's possible to piece your life back together and open up your heart to all of your emotions when you can.

Everyone needs moments of respite from the heaviness of grief and we all need a little joy in life to heal and survive.

Grief doesn't have to be an either-or experience. Keep searching for the "and." It's there even if it's not always easy to find.

Legacy
and Love

Losing someone you love isn't just about missing them. It's about missing the small and most ordinary of things. Things that made your relationship special and all of the things you shared. Things that your loved one is missing out on and should be here to enjoy with you.

—————————————

After the death of someone you love, the missing is unquenchable. Nothing can replace them or completely fill the hole in your heart or the void in your life.

It hurts and it's a journey I wouldn't wish on anyone. Yet losing people we love happens every day and every single person on this earth will come to know the pain of grief. If you're reading this, I'm guessing you know this pain and my heart aches for you.

For anyone who has not experienced the death of a loved one, it's difficult to understand the anguish of missing someone so much it hurts your mind, body, and heart.

You will miss your loved one for the rest of your life. But there are so many other things you will miss as life moves forward and they are no longer here to share it with you.

Their laugh. The sound of their voice. Daily phone calls. The warm hugs only they could give. Sharing a morning cup of coffee. Going out to dinner. Bath time or school holiday parties. Watching your favorite show together on Netflix.

Walking the dog. Sitting on the deck on a warm summer night or making angels in the fresh fallen snow. Reading stories at bedtime. Holding hands. Sharing a beautiful and gentle kiss. Watching them play football or dance at the high school prom.

Grocery shopping and cooking a delicious meal. Going on an unforgettable trip. Taking a drive on a Sunday afternoon. Going to the park. Sharing a lazy rainy day and taking a much-needed nap together.

It's the little things that matter and it's the little things people end up missing the most. There are so many beautiful, unforgettable things that we come to know, look forward to, and experience with those we love. Things we long to see, hear, touch, and do again. But we can't.

It's awful, really, and so hard to accept.

But thank God for the memories. The pictures. The saved voicemails. The stories. The love.

No one can take any of those things away from you, because love is deeply embedded in your soul and heart.

Do something today that will honor your loved one's memory. Wear their sweatshirt. Listen to their favorite song. Go for a Sunday drive to a place you used to go. Plant flowers. Cook a favorite meal or go to that one special coffee shop.

Spread the pictures out on the floor or watch the sacred videos you've taken over the years. Wear a piece of their jewelry or sleep with their favorite stuffed animal.

Pay it forward in their honor by giving back or volunteering.

There are so many things you can do to remember, honor, and keep their legacy front and center in the world.

I know it's hard, and yes, there will be times when doing things that remind you of everything you've lost will feel too painful and will tug at your heart. That's understandable and it's okay if you have moments when the only thing you can do is miss them.

I wish loss wasn't part of being human and I wish the pain of grief never found its way to you. I would give you a hug in person if I could and I hope this book brings you a sense of comfort, validation, and support.

It's normal to focus on the painful
reality that your loved one died,
but it's equally as important to
remember that they lived and
mattered in this life. And the truth
is, your loved one will continue to
live on through you because of all
the beautiful memories carefully
stitched with love into your heart.

Following the death of someone you care about and love, a deep and unfathomable void plants itself in your heart. A void that quickly takes center stage in your life. It's hard to focus on anything but their death and there will be times when it's the only thing you want to think about.

Missing someone you love hurts and the ache runs deep and wide. Perhaps it feels like your mind is stuck on repeat as you ruminate about the day your loved one died. The painful details play over and over again. Details you don't want to remember but never want to forget.

In the early days of grief, it's difficult to concentrate and the magnetic pull of grief is powerful regardless of what you are doing or how busy you are. Whether you want it to or not, grief tends to lurk in the corners of your mind and it's tough to ignore.

It can take a long time for the unthinkable to sink in, and your heart and brain may struggle to believe your loved one is really gone.

I'm not going to sugarcoat my words or pretend the journey of grief is easy. In some ways, grieving the death of a loved one can feel like torture. A kind of torture no one deserves. But grieving is necessary and while it's hard to focus on anything but all that feels so broken, it's important to remember all the things that are not broken in your life too.

One of the things that can help to absorb the aftershocks of loss is to focus on how your loved one lived.

While bittersweet, it's helpful to shift your attention toward remembering all the amazing things that made your beloved so special. Cling to the memories forever stitched into your heart with love.

Remembering and honoring their life is how your loved one lives on through you. While there may always be sadness and grief, the memories can also bring you great joy.

As you relearn how to live life after loss, one of the best ways to honor your loved one is to live in a way that honors the best parts of who they were.

Share their legacy with the world. Share pictures, say their name, and talk about them every single day. Remind the world your loved one will never be forgotten. Remind everyone your loved one mattered and was here.

You will never forget their smile or the way they held your hand. You will never forget their contagious laugh or the way they could lift you up when you were feeling down. You will never forget the way they could light up a room or how deeply they loved you. You will never forget all the things that made them unique or how they made you feel.

There are a million big and little things you will miss for the rest of your life but holding the memories close and honoring their legacy will keep you connected in separation. Love never dies.

Don't let the rules of society drag you down or away from your grief. Don't change one thing about how you need to grieve and never hide your grief from anyone.

Your loved one mattered and the life they lived left an undeniable and beautiful footprint on your soul that doesn't need to be forgotten or hidden away.

It's up to you to bring their memory forward as you find ways to press on. Be the things you loved most about them and they will live on through you. Choose to live life in a way that would make your loved one proud.

There's nothing more beautiful than that, especially when it brings a smile instead of pain and tears. No amount of time will erase the deep grief or love stitched into your heart. But that's the way it's supposed to be when someone you love dies.

When grief feels too heavy, remember how they lived.

Grief is an extension of the love you shared, the love you still feel, and the love that will last forever after losing someone that means more than anything else in your world.

We grieve for so many reasons, but one of the biggest reasons is because of love. It really is that simple and yet grief is one of the most complicated experiences any of us will face in life.

Grief is, without question, messy. When grief settles into the hollowed-out shell of your life, nothing looks familiar and everything feels turned inside out.

But grief is one of the only things that makes sense after death blows up your life.

Grief is here for a reason and it shows up and makes itself at home in our hearts because of love.

Where you find love, you will find grief. They are humbly intertwined in so many ways and both are necessary and important parts of life.

If you really think about it, grief is an extension of the love you will carry for the rest of your days after losing someone you will never forget and always love.

Grief is a powerful and beautiful testament to the strength and endurance of love. Love always stands the test of time and both will continue to live on and be ever present long after your loved one is gone.

I know these are just words and I understand that knowing the reason behind the grief we carry doesn't make it easier right now. I know love doesn't completely take your pain away. The journey of grief will be one of the most difficult journeys you will take.

Loss hurts, but in most cases it hurts because of love. The grief you've been asked to carry is heavy and there will be times when you feel like you might break if you're asked to carry anything more.

On those difficult days, grab on tight to that love and don't let go. Hold on to the good memories and let the love sustain you and carry you through this dark season of your life.

No one can take love away from you. In some ways, grief keeps us connected to our loved ones because it walks hand in hand with all the love overflowing from our hearts.

It's my hope the love you hold deep in your heart will bring you less pain and more joy today.

You won't let your loved one down.
You will never forget them or leave
them behind. They were bigger than
life, and they will always be bigger
than death. You will love them and
honor them for the rest of your days.

———————————

I'm always shocked when society expects a griever to get over the death of a loved one and move on.

If you really think about it, that makes no sense.

We are born to love and connect with others. There are people in our lives whom we love so deeply that life is just better because of them.

We love hard and when one of those special people dies, we will grieve hard.

There is no forgetting someone you love.

There is no getting over losing them or completely moving on from a loss that disrupted your life and turned your heart inside out.

There is no leaving your loved one behind.

Love doesn't die or fade away even as time takes you farther away from the day you last saw them or had to say goodbye.

The people we love often feel bigger than life, and yes, they can feel bigger than death too.

Of course you will always love them, honor them, talk about them, grieve for them, and miss them for the rest of your life.

That's how love, life, and death are meant to be—don't let anyone tell you otherwise.

You get to say their name, honor them, and grieve for them

without guilt or shame. You get to because you are human and you had the gift of loving someone deeply, knowing they loved you back.

I will never let my loved ones down. I will always love and honor their legacies. I will continue to talk about them and live my life trying to mirror the things I loved about them the most. I do it to remind the world they mattered and they were here.

Grief will bring sadness and pain but when intertwined with love, both can help you to stay connected to your loved one, and their legacy will live on because of you.

No one will completely understand the depth of your grief because they can't possibly know the depth of your love for the person you will miss for the rest of your life. Both love and grief are deeply connected and both will remain forever in your heart.

———————————

Sometimes it's really hard to understand why society struggles to show up with compassion when it comes to loss and grief. It's true that people are generally uncomfortable with grief but I think it runs deeper than that.

As sad as it is, we live in a society that often fears death and when the people in your life see your grief and pain, it's a reminder that awful things do happen in life, and it could happen to them. It feels safer to ignore your pain because the rest of the world doesn't want to think about it or think about the price we pay for love.

We grieve, in part, because we are vulnerable enough to love, and love is one of life's greatest gifts. The greater the love, the greater the grief. But the love shared and the love you feel for the special people in your life is personal and sacred to you. Every relationship is unique and different, and it's impossible for anyone else to truly grasp the depth of love and the attachment you had with your loved one.

When someone you love dies, it delivers a soul-crushing blow. The pain is like no other and the grief that settles into your heart is one of the heaviest things you will ever be asked to carry. And while love is a beautiful gift, love is also a source of our pain.

Both love and grief will ask a lot of you, but love doesn't wrap you in Teflon and shield you from loss and pain. Its role isn't to protect you from the awful things that happen in life; it is here to provide comfort and help to carry you through the most difficult of times.

No one can possibly know and understand the depth of your grief because they don't know or understand the love you shared with others in life or the love you continue to carry after death.

Both love and grief are personal to you and both will always have a special place in your heart. No amount of time can steal that from you.

If love remains, the grief will remain—in most cases, for the rest of your life. Love and grief are bundled together as a package deal and both will travel with you wherever you go. Both are a testament to how much you miss someone long after they are gone.

No one should have to carry the deep pain that comes with loss, and I will never diminish or minimize how dreadful any of this is for you.

And there's nothing anyone can do or say that will take your heartache away. People won't necessarily understand your grief because they can't possibly understand how deep the love you carry runs, but at the end of the day, the only one it needs to make sense to is you.

The truth is, you will live, you will love, and you will lose. But love and grief were never meant to be confined, and experiencing both to the fullest is part of what it means to be human.

Give yourself grace today and give the gift of grace to anyone who wants to be there for you but can't possibly understand.

And when it feels like you have nothing else to hold on to, hold on to love as tightly as you can.

Sometimes grief brings comfort to our broken hearts because it's one of the strongest links in the chain that keeps you connected to the person you love long after they are gone.

Grief is so hard and it hurts. No one gets to escape from the experience of grieving, and honestly, when the magnitude of a life-changing loss seems to destroy everything around you, grief is one of the only things that makes sense.

We grieve because we love and where you find one you will find the other.

So when people tell me they are afraid to move forward in life when grieving, I get it. People fear that if their grief softens or the intensity begins to fade, so too will the memories and the love.

It can feel confusing when the sharp edges of grief dull. The conflicting emotions that begin to emerge and reveal themselves can lead to hesitation and guilt.

Some people will desperately cling to the sides of their grief as if it's an unsinkable life raft keeping them afloat. People don't want to surrender to joy or hope because they fear losing connection with their beloved in a world transformed by loss.

There was a time when I felt safer with and comforted by my grief. I knew how to be a sad grieving person, and grief had become my trusted companion, a friend I could count on to be there for me every day. I felt grounded by the pain and knew what to expect even though it was hard.

Sometimes it became an excuse to stay home. To remain adrift in a sea of sadness, guilt-free and alone. I believed grief kept me better connected to my loved one and I was afraid to let that go. If my grief softened, I would forget the things I loved about them most. And honestly, I didn't want to do the hard work it was going to take to move forward and fit back into the world.

Can you relate?

It's true grief becomes part of your daily routine and for a very long time, grief is one of the only things that feels familiar. As strange as it sounds, grief sometimes provides an extra layer of warmth in a world that can feel so dark and cold.

When grief moves in, it shapes and molds parts of who you are and who you will become. So it's easy to question who you are if you're no longer engulfed in sadness or holding daily vigils to keep your grief center stage as you carefully step forward into the unknown.

I understand it's confusing, but inevitably, there will be people who find comfort in the pain.

However, it's important to remember your loved one's memory doesn't live in the pain of your grief. Their legacy and what made them unforgettable lives deep within your heart. You may always grieve, and you may always be a little bit sad, but grief doesn't have to define everything about you, your identity, or who you will become.

Undeniably, grief is and will always be a powerful testament to the love you carry for your loved one. And it is one link in the chain that keeps you connected to the love you shared before and the love that remains long after they are gone.

Grief is proof you are forever connected to your loved one even though their absence has left a big hole in your heart.

So I know it can feel unnerving and scary as you slowly begin to heal and it might seem like you are leaving your loved one behind as you learn to move forward in life.

But you're not leaving them behind. You will never forget and you will discover ways to bring your loved one and all the memories forward into your new and different world. Love never dies and it will never leave you or your grief's side.

Grieving doesn't mean you're sentenced to a lifetime of anguish and despair. And there's a big difference between carrying grief and suffering every day.

You may always grieve, but you don't have to suffer for the rest of your life. You deserve to move forward and find a safe place to grieve and thrive at the same time. You deserve to be happy and to find purpose in your life again.

Remember, even if grief softens, you will never forget and you won't leave your loved one behind.

Grief is the heart's way of letting the world know that you have been asked to live life without someone you love more than anything in the world by your side. Someone you will always miss and who can never be replaced. Your grief is a sacred and personal testament of love and you should never feel pressured to hide it from anyone.

Grief often gets a bad rap. Society treats grief as if it's a taboo subject, and sadly, it's often ignored. People feel awkward around grief and, instead of supporting the grieving, they constantly try to silence it and push it away.

Honestly, it's hard for me to accept the views of a grief-illiterate society. Grief is a natural and normal part of life. Grief is something that everyone will experience, so why is it so difficult to talk about and accept?

There's an infestation of unspoken grief and it's hurting everyone. Efforts to silence it only make the grief experience harder. If pain is repressed, it will unfold and unravel in ways that inevitably can make everything feel worse.

The pain that comes with losing a loved one is incredibly difficult to carry, but grief has meaning and serves an important purpose after a devastating loss.

Grief isn't like an old piece of art hidden away in the attic, forgotten and left alone to gather dust. Grief is valuable and it's meant to be appreciated and experienced.

Following a heartbreaking loss, grief doesn't hesitate to settle deep inside the wounds of your heart. I have always thought of grief as the heart's valiant effort to stay connected to the many loved ones we lose over the years.

Grief is the heart's way of holding a loved one close while honoring the mark they left in the world long after they are gone. It's the heart's way of showing the world just how deeply you love and miss someone.

And that's a beautiful thing.

You should never feel ashamed of your grief or feel pressured to hide it away collecting dust. Grieving is a necessary and human part of your personal journey and sometimes grief is meant to stay.

Still, grief doesn't expect you to stay trapped in the rubble of pain forever, nor are you sentenced to a lifetime of suffering. Grief doesn't forbid anyone from finding moments of joy and happiness, and when you're ready, you can dig your way out of the rubble and good moments will come. How your grief looks today will be very different from how it looks down the road.

Grief is willing to share the space inside your heart. It's not an either-or kind of thing.

I know your heart aches, and on those days when the missing runs deep through your bones, I'm guessing you hate knowing grief at all. I wish grief didn't hurt as much as it does but things will become more tolerable, and as you carry grief forward, remember it's here for a reason. Remember it's the heart's way of reminding you love never ends.

Conclusion

I must admit I struggled with how to finish this book. There are so many important topics to talk about when it comes to loss and grief, and it's impossible to cover everything in a book.

With that being said, I tried to write about things that matter. I hope this book has made a difference for you and anyone who personally knows the pain of grief.

The truth is, there are no perfect words. Nothing I write will bring you complete closure or take your grief away.

I don't have all the answers, which can make it challenging to write about a topic that everyone experiences differently and in their own unique way. I realize that some of what I wrote here in this book may feel relatable to you and there will be other things I shared that completely miss the mark.

That's because grief isn't a one-size-fits-all experience. It's impossible for me to know your personal life experiences, relationships, losses, or where you're at in your own grief journey, but it's my hope you found validation and comfort in some of the pages of this book.

I hope you feel less alone after having read it. Remember that while certain chapters may not resonate with you today, they may bring you comfort down the road.

It would be easier to write about rainbows and gratitude. To encourage you to look at the bright side and try to cheer you up. But I've learned plastering positivity over the pain of grief rarely works.

As difficult as it is, I believe you have to be willing to walk through the pain and not around it. It's important to feel all your emotions and give yourself permission to grieve. It's a long, hard journey and it's not for the faint of heart.

If the loss is big enough, you will most likely grieve for the rest of your life. Even years later, the most ordinary of moments can trip you up and lead to an emotional meltdown. And that's okay. Losing someone or something you love will hurt for a long time.

I don't like to sugarcoat things when it comes to how challenging grief really is, but this book wouldn't be complete without offering encouragement and hope. It's important for you to remember it's possible to live a good and full life again.

You may always feel a little bit sad; after all, there are some things in life that can't be replaced. You will always miss your loved one and you may always yearn for what was.

But the grief you carry will soften, and it won't always feel as painful or intense. It takes time, patience, and grace—grace for yourself and grace for a world that doesn't always get it or understand your pain.

Remember, pain is inevitable after a heartbreaking loss but suffering is optional. And even if you grieve forever, that doesn't mean the pain has to last forever. As much as loss sucks, it can be a catalyst for making deeper connections, finding a renewed sense of purpose, and sometimes, for much-needed change.

Life will be different, but the fog will lift and it's possible to find hope, joy, and meaning again.

I love the Japanese art of kintsugi, which is all about putting broken pottery pieces back together with gold. Kintsugi is built on the idea that through embracing imperfections and flaws, you can create a piece of art that is even stronger, more resilient, and more beautiful than the original.

Every single break is unique and instead of repairing an item to look like new, this process highlights the scars as part of the design. It's a lovely metaphor for healing ourselves when everything feels so unrecognizable and broken. Sometimes through the process of repairing our broken hearts, we can actually create something unique, beautiful, and resilient with time. It is possible to rebuild in the midst of imperfection, and even though you may always carry grief and life may never look quite the same, you can slowly patch the broken pieces back together—scars and all.

While you may feel like your life is in ruins, you can rise above the wreckage and slowly rebuild. It may be difficult to see the road ahead but the ruins we experience in life can transform people in the most profound ways.

This book was written for you with heart and grit. I wouldn't have been able to write any of it if not for a collection of losses and cumulative grief of my own over the years. This book wouldn't be possible if I had not experienced love, pain, and grief. And as hard as the journey of grief has been, I have found ways to rise above the ruins and live a full life again.

And so can you.

I'm hoping you can find the courage to face directly into the storms that may be brewing in your heart. Whether you feel like it or not, you're a brave, amazing human being and you're more resilient than you think. I'm rooting for you.

Don't give up. Have faith that life can be beautiful again even though it won't be the same as it was before. I'm proud of you and encourage you to reach for love when you're having a hard day. You loved before loss found its way into your heart and you will continue to love today, tomorrow, and beyond. Thankfully, love is bigger than death and love never ends. And remember, you yourself are not broken; your heart is.

Thank you for honoring your grief and reading this book. My heart will continue to stand in solidarity with yours and I'm always sending you light and love.

With deep gratitude and love,
Michele

Acknowledgments

I have learned relationships are so important in life, and when grieving a difficult loss, the gifts of connection, companionship, and support are vital to our well-being. And for me, the love and support from family, friends, colleagues, and fellow grievers while writing this book were invaluable from start to finish.

This book wouldn't have been possible if not for so many people I love and value in my life, and I'm beyond grateful to each and every one of you.

My dear mom was my biggest fan. Thank you, Mom, for believing in this book and for encouraging me to follow this dream. I miss you beyond words and wish you could be here to hold this book in your hands. We did it, Mom. I love you.

To my husband, Neal—you are my rock and I truly appreciate all your love, support, and generosity in life. And on those days I wanted to quit, thank you for your encouragement and for giving me the space I needed to lose myself in the writing that is part of who I am. I love you and I'm grateful for us every single day.

To all of our kids—you are all beautiful souls and you have blessed our lives with so much love and joy. Life is better with you in it, and I'm so grateful I get to call you mine. You continue to inspire me, and I'm so proud of your heart and determination to make this world a better place. Keep shining. I love you.

To my sweet grandchildren—I didn't know I could feel so much joy, and my heart is full. Thank you for the laughter, hugs, and unconditional love. Mimi loves you, and you inspire me to be the best I can be every day. May you grow up and carry my heart with you always.

To my family and friends—thank you for showing up for me when life is hard and for your unwavering support throughout this process. Your love and encouragement kept me going on those difficult days when I couldn't seem to find the words. I'm fortunate to have such amazing people in my life, and there isn't a day that goes by when I'm not grateful for you. I love you all.

To my mentors and the wonderful people I have met along the way who do this sacred work—I have learned so much from each of you. You continue to inspire me with your grace, compassion, and wisdom as you fight to make a difference in the world. It's an honor to share this space with you.

To my dear fellow grievers—your heart, grace, courage, vulnerability, and compassion continue to touch my heart and inspire me every day. You remind me why I do this work; you are the reason I wrote this book. Keep fighting your way forward. You deserve to find joy and peace in your life again. I'm so proud of you.

To the Wise Ink team—thank you for walking with me through every step of this process and believing in this book. Your insights, direction, and guidance were invaluable, and I couldn't think of a better team to collaborate with. Thank you for helping me to bring this book out into the world.

About the Author

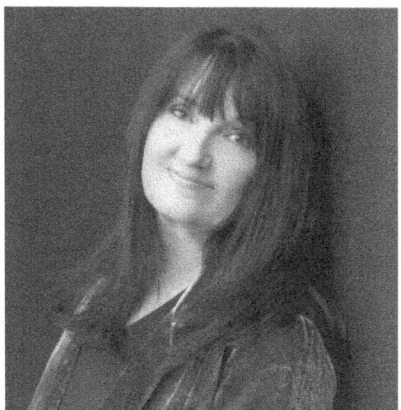

Michele DeVille is a grief specialist, educator, speaker, and coach who seeks to create a safe place for anyone experiencing the devastation of loss. She holds degrees in psychology and communications, several grief support certifications, and also draws expertise and compassion from her own experiences with heartbreaking loss.

Beyond her passion for coaching, speaking, and facilitating grief-support groups, Michele has also fostered a digital community through her popular Instagram and Facebook pages. She regularly shares reminders and affirmations to her base of more than forty thousand people. Her second book, *Your Loss Matters*, is helping her support and reach more hearts—offering tangible comfort to the grief community.

To get Michele's free self-care guide and learn more about her services, visit her online at **MicheleDeVille.com**.